CONTENTS

KT-442-234

Raising Voices: Ensuring Quality in Residential Care

An Evaluation of the Caring in Homes Initiative

P. J. Youll & C. McCourt-Perring

Brunel University 1993

London: HMSO

ISBN 0 11 321630 0

The Authors

Penny Youll, is a Senior Research Fellow at Brunel University and was Director of the Coordination and Evaluation Group of the Caring in Homes Initiative. Christine McCourt-Perring is a Research Fellow at Brunel University and worked full time for the Coordination and Evaluation Group.

FOREWORD

It is not an overstatement to assert, as this book does, that it both raises a series of fundamental questions and highlights serious issues that will shape the provision of residential care in the future. Traditional notions of residential care are beginning to change, but real change will only come if these questions and issues are discussed and debated in a wider forum. 'Raising Voices' has given a strong lead, speaking with authority and openness.

The longer I read this most important contribution to the debate on residential care, the more certain I feel that a successor body to the Wagner Development Group needs to be set up to take forward so many of the issues and ideas discussed on these pages.

For instance, the Caring in Homes Initiative was set up to help to promote and ensure the quality of life of people living in care homes—yet 'reaching residents was a challenge and one which we failed to meet as adequately as we wished'. And again, 'It was their sadness or quiet anger or sense of powerlessness that reached through their measured and polite words; it was these feelings that helped us to recognise the importance of what they were saying'.

Given the difficulty of involving residents, the success of Inside Quality Assurance (IQA) in making user views central to the review makes the need to give IQA external validation seem vital. Managers and proprietors look for formal recognition and this is to be welcomed, as is the use of BS 5750 in that it shows a widespread desire to improve practice, but the merits of IQA need to be more widely known to help tilt the balance in favour of residents' involvement.

The CHI work also clearly highlights the benefits of residents and staff being more involved in thinking about the developments that need to take place. In this respect, the work on training and on making links with local communities show new ways forward. Similarly, providing appropriate and useful information for residents and their carers emerges as an essential task in service provision—the work of CHI shows that this is a key aspect of ensuring quality.

Specialised care provision has placed greater emphasis on meeting people's physical and age related needs but the CHI has highlighted the importance of looking at needs from a generic point of view and the high value placed on meeting emotional and social needs of residents.

There has been nothing to compare with the depth and breadth of the research this very important review has set out to assess. I have mentioned but a few of the many important issues it has addressed. Statutory and voluntary agencies lack knowledge of how to involve users, how to set up effective consultation or how to set up structures for participation. The CHI programme guidelines provide ideas and practice-based approaches for taking these aspects forward and I commend 'Raising Voices' to all who wish to see residential care as a positive choice for all those who use it and for the staff who run the services.

Gillian Wagner

ACKNOWLEDGEMENTS

The Caring in Homes Initiative was commissioned and funded by the Department of Health. We wish to record our warm appreciation of the encouragement received from Cyril Stone and his successor Anne de Peyer and the considerable support provided by Simon Hiller throughout the research. Our discussions at the Department of Health also included valuable help from the Research Management Division originally from Madeleine Sims and latterly from Ruth Chadwick. We also wish to thank Lionel Harrison and Judith Downey from the SSI for their interest and the contributions they made to our thinking.

Our greatest debt of gratitude is to all those who, for reasons of confidentiality, we are unable to name and thank personally. We are enormously grateful to the residents, their relatives and carers, volunteers, care staff, home managers and proprietors and the senior managers who we met and who gave their time to talk with us. We realise that, for nearly everyone, we were approaching them at a difficult and worrying time. For many, being asked to comment was a new experience and not always a comfortable one: we especially appreciate the courage it took for some people to talk with us at all. We believe that the courtesy and interest with which we were received says much for the intrinsic importance of the CHI work and the general willingness of all those involved to look ahead and make changes. Without these contributions this evaluation would have few useful outcomes. In many ways, as this book will show, the CHI is the result of the work and thinking of people living and working in residential establishments. We hope this account does justice to their experience.

As evaluators we were dependent on the goodwill and support of our CHI colleagues in the agencies commissioned to conduct the developmental research. This book provides us with the opportunity to thank them for their generous co-operation with a complicated research programme which involved all of us in a wide variety of contacts across project sites and agencies. We learnt much from their wide experience and valued highly the discussions and debates we shared. We particularly want to mention those with whom we worked most closely:

Leonie Kellaher, Diane Willcocks, Sheila Peace, Maggie Veitch and Sue Lawrence at the Centre for Environmental and Social Studies of Ageing, University of North London;

Nick Moore, Jane Steele, Ian Rowlands, Sean Roberts, Chris Dawson and Alice Bloch at the Policy Studies Institute;

Des Kelly and Kate Freeman at the Social Care Association (Education) and project consultants John Burton, Tom Hanchen, Micki Lovell, Charles Pragnell and Vicky White;

Chris Payne at the National Institute for Social Work and project consultants, Steve Brooks, Colin Kelcey, George Mabon, Tina Miller, Liz Peretz, Julia Phillipson, Vanessa Wiseman, Keith Woods.

The CHI was represented on the Post Wagner Development Group and special thanks are due its members for their interest and highly informed advice. The Group provided an invaluable forum for debate of crucial issues: the working groups, the support and critical commentaries from individual members all added greatly to our understanding of the contemporary scene. We must give particular thanks to Gillian Wagner who chaired the Group from 1990 and who has been so unfailingly energetic in championing developments in residential care: the CHI was no exception.

We are especially grateful to a number of people for sharing with us information and views and giving advice. Our interviews with people in specialised agencies were particularly important in giving us an understanding of services from the points of view of different care groups, carers, users and consumers. Their willingness to give time to the interviews helped immeasurably to establish the resident focus of the evaluation: we hope that we have done justice to the wealth of ideas and observations they provided. Unfortunately, it is not possible to thank every one individually but the organisations and agencies they represented are listed in Appendix 2: to all we extend our warm thanks.

We would like to record our gratitude to Bandana Ahmad, of the Race Equality Unit NISW, who gave us good counsel and advice on formulating a set of statements and guidelines on anti-discriminatory practice.

We are grateful too to all those who contributed to seminars and workshops, including students at Brunel on the Masters course in Public and Social Administration and the MPhil in Social Work: their observations and criticisms were informed and stimulating.

At Brunel we owe thanks most of all to Maurice Kogan and Mary Henkel, our colleagues and friends, who acted as consultants to the team and worked with us throughout. Without their experience, knowledge and considerable support we would have been less able to encompass the tasks and unable to retain a critical overview of the CHI.

Other colleagues in CEPPP have also been generous in their help: we would like to thank in particular Christopher Pollitt, Martin Cave, Sandra Jones, Richard Joss and Val Beale. We are indebted to those who worked with us on parts of the evaluation: we are grateful to Deborah Rutter and Marilyn Kirk for their hard work and stimulating contributions and to

Sophie Aindow, a student on placement, who worked with enthusiasm and efficiency. David Mathers was of great assistance with computing matters: to him our thanks.

While acknowledging the considerable contribution that others have made to our work and thinking we remain entirely responsible for the way we have interpreted the information we gathered and for the ideas and views expressed.

Our final thanks go to Sally Harris. She administered the work with exemplary efficiency, kept track of us as we toured the country, helped to organise our seminars and conferences and generally provided a home base for the team. Like others before us, we relied on Sally's speed and accuracy in producing drafts of the book. For these skills we are grateful indeed. But our special thanks are for her interest and commitment to the work: the issues involved in residential care touched her as they have so many of us.

Penny Youll and
Christine McCourt-Perring
Brunel University
August 1993

PART ONE

The Caring in Homes Initiative in Context

Chapter 1

THE CARING IN HOMES INITIATIVE

This book is an account and an evaluation of a major programme of developmental research in residential care practice and management—the Caring in Homes Initiative (CHI).

It addresses a series of fundamental questions about residential care and services in the nineties and highlights issues that will shape the provision of care into the next century.

The central issue—the organising theme of the Initiative—was to promote quality of life for those who live in a residential care establishment, however long or short their stay; whatever their situation, age, ability; whatever their background, race or culture.

The CHI is particularly important for two reasons.

It focused on the needs and concerns of those who live and work in residential care homes: the work was conducted in individual establishments in collaboration with frontline staff, care home managers and proprietors and residents. Over 260 homes and agencies took part in projects across the country. The experience, perceptions and commentaries of people at the grassroots revealed a need for a reappraisal of our traditional notions of residential care, of the need for and purposes of care, of the priorities for change and development, of approaches to management and to training. Above all, they demonstrated that residents can participate and be involved in the way services are run and developed.

Second, the Initiative looked at residential accommodation and service provision across the board. This was the first time a major research programme had worked on a generic basis: the projects included all the main care groups. The importance of this has increased as the implementation of community care has proceeded. The work showed that the different groupings have much to learn from each other and that the common needs and interests of those living in residential homes outweigh the differences. Again, the work highlighted the scope for new thinking about how people's needs are defined and responded to.

These features—the grassroots and generic nature of the CHI—have led to a deeper appreciation of the tasks of residential services, why they are needed, how care homes need to be integrated within the range of care services in the community and how residents and their carers, together with staff and managers, have key roles and responsibilities in service development and quality assurance.

The Caring in Homes Initiative was a three-year programme commissioned by the Department of Health in 1989 to demonstrate how some of the recommendations of the Wagner review on residential care (Wagner, 1988) might be implemented. Underpinning these recommendations was an explicit set of values and principles for practice which, in turn, informed the work of the CHI. The central aim was to develop approaches to practice that would help to promote and ensure quality of life of people living in care homes.

The Initiative comprised the following Programmes of research and development:

Inside Quality Assurance: Internal Review for Residential Homes— run by the Centre for Environmental and Social Studies of Ageing, the University of North London (CESSA). The aim was to develop ways of enabling the individual care establishment to carry out in-house reviews that involved residents and frontline staff;

Window in Homes: Links Between Residential Establishments and the Community—run by the Social Care Association (Education) (SCA). The aim was to explore how care homes could establish and benefit from closer links with their local community and enable residents to be more involved;

Information for Users of Personal Social Services—run by the Information Policy Unit of the Policy Studies Institute (PSI). The aim was to describe ways of providing residents and potential service users with information as a means of enhancing choice. The Programme also conducted an additional piece of work on *Information about Residential Care for Elderly People*;

Training for Care Workers—run by the National Institute for Social Work (NISW). The aim was to develop approaches and tools for in-house training that would enhance the understanding and care practice of basic level staff.

In addition to these, a fifth agency was commissioned:

Co-ordination and Evaluation Group—based in the Centre for Evaluation of Public Policy and Practice, Brunel University (C & E Group). The tasks were to co-ordinate the work of the CHI, to conduct an evaluation of the Programmes as they progressed and to provide an independent appraisal of the Initiative as a whole. This book is the result of that work.

The work of the Initiative was wide ranging and ambitious. It was undertaken during a period of unprecedented policy change in community-based care services and a high level of public and professional concern about care standards. The development Programmes were working at a time of anxiety and uncertainty—particularly for people working at the grassroots who are not, usually, those in a good position to understand the broad picture of change and its implications. It was a climate which created difficulties for the researchers but at the same time helped to highlight key issues and may also have led to greater receptivity to change on the part of the practitioners and care agencies involved.

There were several features of the CHI which it is helpful to outline at the outset.

First of all it was concerned with translating principles of good practice and broad statements of policy into workable and useful ideas and approaches. The work was determined by the recommendations of the Wagner review which set the rights and needs of the resident as the central values for service provision, development and review. The whole tenor of the work was about learning from those most directly involved in providing and using services in order that the guidelines and materials produced would be effective and relevant. The developments were, therefore, shaped more by consumer and frontline experience than broad organisational objectives or strategic plans.

Second, the work encompassed a range of interests. By working with all the main care groups and the different sectors of provision, the CHI researchers were concerned with multiple perspectives—those of residents, frontline staff, providers, carers and families. The Programmes were involved not only in understanding these interests and views but also the significance of different, divergent or conflicting approaches to meeting residents' needs and aspirations.

Third, the Initiative was a complex and multi-layered programme. Although the overall aims and purposes were the same in each case, Programmes worked independently, set up projects and developed their approaches in a variety of ways. This diversity led to some difficulty in recognising and appreciating the common ground between the Programmes during the course of the research. But part of the strength of the CHI lies in a strong convergence both in the overall picture of residential life and work to emerge and in the approaches to quality practice which resulted.

Lastly, the work was to be innovative and to learn from working in collaboration with ordinary care homes and agencies. The homes which participated were not selected because they were special in any particular way: they included establishments which were experiencing problems as well as those which were seeking to make improvements to the quality of the service or to involve residents more fully. Definitions of good practice, of quality of life and quality of service and ideas about how to implement them were, therefore, explored directly with practitioners and, wherever possible, residents themselves.

These features set in place particular challenges for the four agencies concerned and these will be discussed as we look at the work of each Programme.

Evaluating the Initiative

Evaluation was central to the work of the CHI and in three main ways:

- *self-evaluation* was expected to be an integral part of the developmental work of each Programme.

- the C & E Group was responsible for a *formative evaluation* based on working alongside the researchers, observing project activities and carrying out fieldwork in the participant homes and agencies. The Group provided informal feedback during the work and two reviews of each Programme.

- *a summative evaluation* of the Initiative as a whole was also conducted by the C & E Group. This was to provide an independent set of judgements about the work overall and an external validation based on studying the way the work was pursued, the materials published and the extent to which the projects resulted in benefits for residents.

Values and approaches

It was important that the evaluation took a stance that was compatible with the values and assumptions on which the CHI was based. Its origins in the Wagner review meant that the primary source of evaluation was that of the service user. But good practice and the maintenance of a high quality of service also rest on staff, on management, on appropriate resources and levels of support. The interests of care staff and managers were important: their views were essential in understanding life and work in the home and how user needs can be met. Equally, the needs of the families and carers of residents impinge on the way residential services are perceived, used and run: their views too, were important.

It was necessary, therefore, to approach any appreciation of the CHI in a pluralist way that allowed multiple interests to be recognised while taking those of the resident—the direct service user—as central. This was done by paying particular attention to the views of those at the grassroots.

There were several justifications for doing so.

Residents are the intended beneficiaries of the service and, as such, their experience and perceptions are central to any assessment of quality. Their welfare is closely connected to those who provide care—often involving staff in intimate physical contact and considerable emotional investment. If staff are disaffected in any way this will affect their relationships with residents.

A different reason comes from the notion that it is people at the bottom of an organisation who see and understand most about how it works and what is really going on. Hartsock suggests that the less dominant 'have to understand and predict the views and attitudes of the more powerful in order to ensure their own survival'.

On the other hand, people in power have a more partial view as

'it is in their interests to reinforce the status quo which continues to legitimate their power' (Hartsock, 1983)

People at the grassroots have a vital interest in retaining their jobs or their home and we quickly recognised the detailed awareness they have of every aspect of residential life. For residents, survival is a real issue: people fear losing their place in an establishment if they do not conform. Their wellbeing—and perhaps survival—depends on knowing how things run, who is in charge, what is acceptable. They were aware of things that management did not see and they expressed different views from those at the top.

We were, then, concerned with making sense of the projects through the experience of those involved. We anticipated that the results would reveal different perceptions, ideas and ideals. We were interested in meanings rather than measurements, with understanding and describing experience rather than gathering objective data (Guba and Lincoln, 1989).

The aims of evaluation

The C & E Group aimed, first, to produce an analytic description of the work of the research teams and a commentary on the authority of the materials developed. This included considering the sources of knowledge and views which contributed to the work, how new approaches were introduced and implemented, how the experience of the projects was refined, formulated and published. Projects were learning about how care establishments might initiate and manage change so the *processes involved*—the interactions and relationships—were important to understand.

The range and diversity of the projects meant that one of the tasks of evaluation was to understand the importance of the different organis-ational, care group and practice *contexts* within which the work was developed: what helps and what hinders the implementation of new approaches?

Second, the Group was asked to comment on the significance of CHI overall. This included looking at the findings across the Programmes and care groups and providing a series of judgements on the potential relevance, benefits and costs of their work based on the outcomes of the developmental projects. The Group did not evaluate the final products of the Programmes' work: these were published as the evaluation work was ending.

The methods used

The nature of the work called for a qualitative approach to evaluation which allowed the contexts of the work, the processes and interactions involved and different viewpoints and interests to be understood.

There were important issues relating to access. Those participating in the projects had to be reassured that the evaluation was not concerned with judgements about their performance or that of their home: it was about gaining information, views and feedback from staff, managers and residents about the research projects. It was essential, therefore, that we took time to negotiate contacts, to be seen to take a neutral, exploratory interest in what was going on and to give opportunities for people to comment, ask questions and check our perceptions and interpretations.

These considerations pointed to a detailed, case study approach and opportunities to work alongside project workers and participants where this was acceptable. We visited the sites—usually care homes—before, during and after the project work to obtain detailed knowledge of the development of the work over time. We talked to the researchers, analysed project and other records, observed and contributed to project activities and meetings, ran discussion meetings ourselves and provided feedback when invited to do so. The work centred, however, on interviews and less formal discussions with the project workers, volunteers, staff, managers and, wherever possible, residents, their relatives and carers. We also interviewed senior managers from the agency concerned with the particular home and from the local SSD in each case study area to gain an overview of the organisational and policy contexts.

However, we also needed to obtain a breadth of coverage so that we had information about work with different kinds of establishment, care groups and sectors. To do so we visited up to ten sites in each Programme and carried out interviews after the end of the project work. We had discussions with a number of consultants from each Programme as well as those involved in the case studies, consulted their records and attended consultant meetings (See Appendix 1).

We also gathered basic data about fifty-five establishments—over half of those involved in the main demonstration projects—as background information about the characteristics of the CHI participants.

To help us understand the issues and priorities for the different care groups and how changes in policy were affecting provision, we visited organisations run for and by service users, relatives and carers and a number of specialised provider agencies (See Appendix 2). The results of this were written up and widely circulated for comment: it was encouraging that we received many responses endorsing and elaborating on the views expressed (Perring 1991).

The hub of the work lay in reaching people most directly concerned with the projects. We wanted people to tell us what was important and what it was like to try out new ideas. We anticipated that many of our respondents would have had little or no experience of being asked to give their views. Ordering one's thoughts in response to someone else's questioning is not an everyday skill. We used semi-structured interviews where possible or guided discussions where this was not appropriate. The aim was to allow people to voice their own ideas and to allow their priorities to come to the fore. This was especially important in relation to residents and frontline staff. Their preoccupations often had little direct relationship to the project in hand. But their comments were crucial in revealing what quality of life meant to them, what constitutes quality care and what helps or hinders good practice.

Reaching residents was a challenge and one which we failed to meet as adequately as we wished. Because we wanted to use unthreatening methods as far as possible, we arranged to spend time informally observing the daily round, having meals, going to the pub, joining in outings, talking with residents' meetings about our work, and generally being with staff and residents (McCourt-Perring 1993). These approaches were generally without difficulty although it was necessary to remind people from time to time that we were not project workers. We learnt much from the way we were introduced to staff and residents and about the way, as outsiders, we were either welcomed or treated with caution.

Reaching residents as individuals was more problematic. There were two main reasons for this. We were unable to arrange to talk to people where care home managers and staff were cautious about agreeing to access: such residents did not have the opportunity to decide for themselves whether or not they wanted to see us. Some degree of protection was, of course, appropriate but we were concerned at the number of times we were told—especially in relation to older people and people with learning disabilities—that residents would have nothing to contribute or that they would not understand. In a few cases this went as far as managers not agreeing to residents being sent a letter explaining who we were and inviting them to participate.

This apparent over protection was in contrast to similar homes— including those for people with particular communication needs—where we were expected to contact residents directly: staff only wanted to know who we were approaching so that they could be on hand to help if needed.

Overall we visited sixty-three homes, across the care groupings, over fifty-five agencies and conducted over 260 formal and semi-formal interviews, including group discussions, with managers, staff and residents.

A brief account of how we analysed the material from this diversity of homes, agencies and range of projects is given in Appendix 3.

The authority of the evaluation

In these ways we built up a picture of the experience and thoughts of a variety of people of all ages and abilities as they sought to improve the quality of service and lifestyle of people in residential care homes. Their ideas and views were focused on the work of CHI but, because of the open-ended nature of our approach to interviews and discussions, not exclusively so. What has emerged, therefore, is not only a commentary and critique of the work of the four Programmes and CHI as a whole, but also a reflection of the contemporary scene in residential services.

Part of the authority of our account and commentary of the Initiative lies in ourselves. We were two full-time researchers who carried out nearly all the fieldwork. We did not specialise: both of us carried out fieldwork in each Programme, all care groupings and types of home. In this way we could each make comparisons, recognise differences and experience the tensions and realities across CHI.

Our evidence also came from the feelings which the work evoked in us—particularly in the care homes we visited. Meeting people living and working in individual establishments was often painful—we were available to listen and people responded. They were not always able to express things directly but their underlying feelings came through. The commentary we make later on the emotional isolation of residents and the anxieties of staff, for example, comes in part from what people said to us. But it was their sadness or quiet anger or sense of powerlessness that reached through their measured and polite words: it was these feelings that helped us to recognise the importance of what they were saying.

In contrast, there were homes where the atmosphere was welcoming and relaxed, people spoke freely and their communications to us were robust: the significant thing was that here the feelings which came across matched the words.

Throughout the work, we took opportunities to discuss our observations and interpretations with our colleagues in the research Programmes, with participants and in specially convened seminars and workshops. One of the most important sources of debate and criticism came from the Post Wagner Development Group on which the C & E Group was represented.

The Way the Book is Organised

We recognise that the CHI covers a wide spectrum of interests and readers may wish to be selective. The book is written, as far as possible, so that the different chapters may be read independently. However, we believe that one of the important lessons of the Initiative is the benefit of looking at practice and development from new perspectives—learning from other care groups, collaborating between sectors, challenging traditions of practice or management or training, taking on board residents' and carers' points of view. We have tried, therefore, to organise the book in such a way that issues like these—which may cut across our usual way of defining and thinking about services—are referred to throughout—even at the risk of some repetition.

In the first part of the book we discuss the origins of the Initiative and the political, organisational, practice and professional contexts within which the work was pursued. The diversity of the field meant that the researchers and evaluators were working with and across a number of different institutions, reference groups, interests and traditions.

The main part focuses on the work of each of the research Programmes in turn. The aim is to give a critical account of how the work was developed, its scope and authority, who was involved, the stages which the research went through, the main factors which shaped the final guidelines and materials and their cost implications. The outcomes of the trial projects and demonstrations are discussed in as far as they are indicative of the potential benefits of the Programmes' work.

The third part takes a cross-Programme look at the lessons to be drawn from the work of the CHI as whole. In Chapter 7 we discuss the contribution they make to understanding the experience of residents and of care staff and how to provide care that meets residents' needs. We go on, in Chapter 8, to discuss issues relating to quality of life—what this means and how it may be promoted. We discuss the notion that a care home should provide an enabling environment—a kind of base camp—from which residents may explore, find fulfilment and establish the lifestyle they prefer. The initiation and management of change—particularly at the grassroots—is discussed as a key aspect of providing services that are responsive and relevant. The CHI raised questions about residential care, the nature of provision, how services are organised and developed and we draw together some ideas about user-led participation in service development and evaluation. The final chapter highlights developmental trends and discusses some of the implications for service providers and users.

Chapter 2

THE CONTEXTS OF RESIDENTIAL SERVICE PROVISION AND DEVELOPMENT

In this chapter we identify the contexts within which the work was developed and discuss, briefly, features that relate to CHI concerns. We do so in order to display the diversity of interests involved and how these impinge on residential care provision. It is also a way of locating the work within policy and practice frames and making reference to some of the main issues and trends.

The Programmes were working in an environment in which they had to take account of a number of institutions, traditions, sources of information, experience and expertise. This meant that the tasks of development and implementation were complex and, because they were carried out at the grassroots, likely to be context specific and strongly shaped by local situations. One of the implications was that each project would be different and that it would be necessary for the researchers to define and understand the specific contexts within which they were working as these related to the individual home, locality and care group involved.

Residential Care in Context

We have identified a number of areas of policy and practice which framed or impinged on the work of the CHI Programmes. These are broadly defined spheres or clusters of interest which it was important to keep in mind:

- *the policy system*: legislation, central policy guidance and practice guidelines, local authority interpretations and implementation arrangements;

- *professional and practitioner interests*: including training systems and agencies, professional associations, recruitment networks, unions and staff associations;

- *providers and the market for residential services*: statutory, voluntary and private agencies, associations of providers, purchasers and fundholders, private consumers;

- *quality assurance, regulatory and monitoring systems;*

- *service user and consumer interests:* user and care group organisations, carers and relatives.

We discuss each of these briefly and focus on those aspects which
presented the researchers with particular challenges.

The Policy System
The policy system includes legislation and centrally defined policies
together with local policy making, planning and implementation.

The broadness of the residential care field means that provision is
subject to a considerable array of legislative frames which apply generally
to the registration, running and regulation of residential care homes as well
as to specific aspects of services—usually relating to particular care
groups.

Policy environment
The period of the research was dominated, however, not by legislation
specifically addressing residential care services, but by the Children Act
1989 and the NHS and Community Care Act 1990 which had major
implications for all residential establishments and provider agencies participating in CHI. Both led to numerous central guidances—the formal
instruments through which the government outlines its requirements for
implementation—and a flood of guidelines—materials providing advice
and information about good practice. The volume of such outputs during
the period and the generally tight timetables for implementation were
without precedent.

In addition to this intense activity, which was radically changing the
contexts within which providers were operating, there were also a series of
enquiries and reports addressing aspects of residential care following
major scandals—mostly in the field of child care (Kahan and Levy, 1991;
Utting, 1991; Warner Report, Department of Health/HMSO, 1992a). The
impact of these was to focus attention onto residential care and to raise
further questions about competence, recruitment, regulation and morale
across the sectors.

One of the crucial issues not recognised at the time—nor since—was
the kind of expertise, the degree of collaboration, the diversity of information and the considerable time scale required to interpret and implement central requirements—especially when coming as thick and fast as
those concerned with community care. It is a strategic management task to
plan and put in place resources and procedures for implementation but, in
the field of personal care services, it is those who work in the front line who
have to take on new arrangements without throwing out good practices
and disrupting essential continuities. The physical and emotional tasks

involved in making sense of the new arrangements, deciding what applies, sorting out priorities and translating everything into a local context were—and for many continue to be—highly stressful.

Policy assumptions

A different set of issues, which we note briefly, concerns the assumptions that underlie central guidelines. These are important in that they strongly influence the way the tasks of providing care are interpreted and how good practice is defined, implemented and monitored.

First, we note the importance of setting out general frames of reference and codes for good practice. Documents like *Homes are for Living In* (DOH/SSI, 1989a) are highly valued—in good part because they are accessible and readable—in helping people to think through crucial issues of practice and provision. One of the most important features is that they try to identify principles as well as define aspects of good practice. There is no doubt that providers and practitioners seek and respond to central guidelines but many do so uncritically.

Second, provision for elderly people still tends to dominate thinking about care services in the community and this is revealed in a number of general materials. The impact of this is, as many of the projects discovered, that guidance assumed to be generic does not meet the particular circumstances of different groups and individuals.

On the other hand, there is an assumption that the different care groups necessarily require separate guidelines on good practice. The main elements in the *Guidance on Standards* series which addresses standards of residential care provision for different care groups (eg DOH/SSI, 1990a, 1990b, 1992a, 1992b) are virtually the same but the distinctions made between groupings reveal stereotypical notions of people's needs and about what is important to them.

Fourth, there is a pervasive tendency to refer to residential services and settings as distinct and apart from care in the community. This is in marked contrast to the assertion made by the Wagner review, and organisations concerned with the provision of services for all care groups, that residential care should be an intrinsic part of the community in which it is located and integrated with other forms of care service.

CHI as policy implementation

As a final comment we should note that the CHI, as a programme commissioned by the government, has its place in the policy system. It was an attempt to influence residential care provision through demonstration and the production of model approaches to practice. It embraced particular values and assumptions—primarily those of the Wagner review—which emphasised the interests of the consumer. In doing so it foreshadowed later government moves to establish the importance of consumer interests, for example, through the publication of the Citizen's Charter.

The impacts of policy development during the period of CHI were, then, considerable. New values were being installed, the place of residential care and the relationship between statutory and independent sectors were being reappraised, care services were moving into a market system: no part of the field was unaffected by the changes.

Professional and Practitioner Interests

The interests of those working in personal care services are based on four main concerns: for secure employment, for career advancement, for professional status and recognition and for quality of service. These are addressed through the institutions and organisational structures which control employment, offer training and qualification, and influence reputation and professional recognition: these span central and local government, professional associations and trade unions.

It has been recognised that residential carers work in an unusual milieu:

'What is specific to group care practice is the context within which workers have to operate ie. working in a semi-public setting in an interdependent team, in a complex network of relationships between team members and users and between individual and group' (para 6.2.2 CCETSW Expert Group 1992).

This means that people's working practice is more on view to peers, more open to criticism, than their field social work counterparts. This level of personal exposure can lead to a heightened sensitivity between staff and between staff and residents. There are obvious concerns, for example, about handling dependency, or the kind of intimate contact required to help some residents, or the level of responsibility for vulnerable young or elderly people. One of the unfortunate—and sometimes disastrous—results of this kind of anxiety is that staff hide what they do: they attempt to tackle problems behind closed doors rather than discuss them with managers or peers. Understanding the nature of a group-based workplace is, then, highly relevant in thinking about quality, practice development and the interests of workers.

The CHI projects were mostly concerned with basic-level and frontline workers. Their interests and identity tended to centre on their particular home and the care group that it served. For many, job satisfaction stemmed from being valued by immediate colleagues and management and by residents but for some—for example in the field of mental health or alcohol recovery work—there was considerable satisfaction from belonging to and being recognised by a specific peer network of practitioners.

The issues relating to the role and provision of training will be discussed in more detail in Chapter 6 where we look at the work of the Training for Care Workers Programme. Here we note the restructuring of basic and post-qualifying training in social work, the development and implementation of a national system of work-based training—the NVQ—the continuing debates about the most effective training for residential care—especially child care and new demands for training coming from community care implementation. The picture is one of considerable turmoil since there are a number of unresolved issues affecting people at every level in residential care provision.

Concerns about secure employment were considerable at a time which brought home closures and organisational restructuring. Changes in the relationship between providing services on the one hand and purchasing according to assessed care needs on the other were creating anxieties for practitioners across the board. People were concerned about personal status and preserving their jobs, their identity and reputation.

Professionals and practitioners are also involved and influential in defining and evaluating what constitutes good practice. Developments in social work and social care practice are shaped by debates within the professional associations and institutions, through practice exchange networks, special interest groups, trade and professional journals and specially constituted bodies like the Post Wagner Development Group (see NISW/HMSO, 1993). However, as with central policy frames, there is a marked tendency for professionals to construct thinking and develop practice within care groups. The CHI research was, therefore, unusual in working across these boundaries. Practitioners identify strongly with the particular care group they serve and this, as we will comment later, has been significant in perpetuating traditional patterns of provision.

Providers and the Market for Services

Provision was undergoing such change during the Initiative that it amounted, for many, to a restructuring of residential services. The relationship and balance between the sectors was changing radically: public sector homes were being closed or floated off as independent companies; private concerns were looking for ways of ensuring their place in the market; voluntary organisations were reviewing their provision. Agencies providing services for care groups not formerly a key responsibility of local authorities—like drug, alcohol, mental health services—were particularly concerned about the level of funding that would be available. Our interviews with people in provider and user organisations revealed similar anxieties across the sectors about funding and financial security, about contracting arrangements, about meeting new demands or finding new customers, about inspection criteria and maintaining quality standards. The main differences were associated less with sector and more with the size of an establishment and whether or not it was part of a wider organisation.

These concerns were not confined to the independent sector: the split between assessment, case management and purchasing on the one hand and the provision of services on the other within social services departments meant that statutory homes were also squaring up to the existence of a market.

The general concerns of providers included:

• many homes in the statutory sector faced the possibility—and realities—of restructuring or closure;

• the development of new funding arrangements and relationships between the provider sectors and fundholders was critical for all. Anxieties about survival in the new market meant that managers and proprietors were having to understand where they stood in relation to potential competitors, contractors and customers;

• people were looking at the possibilities of the emerging market and considering diversification of form and function—for example, resource centres, domiciliary services;

• equally, providers were looking at the potential openings for specialisation—for niches in the market that they might fill;

• providers generally were concerned to maintain quality as the most important way of establishing a reputation in the market place;

• many providers had a mixed attitude to staff training because they feared losing trained workers to field social work, but many saw investment in staff as a key means of ensuring quality of service. However, homes participating in the CHI projects showed a high level of staff stability. Although this sample is not typical it may indicate that there is actually less turnover than used to be the case;

• the restructuring of financial support for residents.

The period during which the CHI was being carried out saw, as a result of these changes, a heightened awareness of other agencies and a shift in emphasis from internal concerns to external relationships. Private and commercial providers were either taking the initiative in forging new contacts with the local authority and other fundholders or being forced to do so. There was an increasing recognition of the importance of knowing and being known in the market place. People were taking on new ideas about, for example, information exchange, reputation building, how to demonstrate quality. This may well have led to a greater willingness to participate in new projects and to learn about new approaches than might otherwise have been the case.

Quality Assurance, Regulatory and Monitoring Systems

Since CHI was commissioned to promote the quality of residents' lives, issues relating to quality assurance, standard setting, the monitoring and regulation of service provision were central to the research. It has been helpful to make distinctions between:

- *quality assurance*—the internal frameworks, procedures and activities which are designed to ensure that a quality service is provided. These are measures set in place by the service provider and are essentially internal, operational systems;

- *quality control*—concerned with monitoring and inspecting services to ensure that they meet both external requirements and regulations and internally set specifications. These activities may be conducted by internal as well as external inspectors.

A further distinction to be made is, then, between internal and external systems. This is helpful in clarifying internal operational responsibilities for ongoing review and development services, for standard setting, service specification and those which are externally framed—by, for example, legal requirements, registration criteria and professional norms and expectations.

The period of CHI saw an increasing emphasis on quality issues. All the agencies and homes involved were aware of the importance of demonstrating the quality of their services. But there was also much confusion about how standards can be measured, about inspection criteria and particularly about the language used in reviewing and monitoring services.

The CHI Programmes were not developing quality assurance systems as such nor were they concerned primarily with quality control. The work aimed to ensure that everyday practice—in training, management, internal and external relationships, information exchange—promoted high quality. As such they were making a contribution to quality assurance.

A key development during the Initiative was the establishment of inspection units. For the first time homes run by the local authority came within the same systems of regulation and inspection as those in the independent sector. This, and the development of the split between purchasers and providers of services, put the spotlight on internal quality assurance, operational responsibilities, systems for setting and monitoring standards and service outputs.

Of particular relevance to CHI work were the following:

- the definition of criteria for inspection and the extent to which these were generic across care groupings. The dominance of SSD personnel in the so-called arm's length units was generating anxiety from providers for care groups which had not been a central part of SSD provision;

- exploring the distinctions between the developmental role of inspection and that of delivering judgements.

Service User and Consumer Interests

Here we distinguish between different groupings of service users and consumers:

- residents who live in establishments;

- organisations, campaign and rights groups promoting the interests of users;

- individuals and the general public who are potential service users;

- the carers and relatives of residents: their needs and interests are different and distinct from those of residents but they are, nonetheless, indirect beneficiaries and users of care services.

Organisations which promote the interests of users include those which are run for and also by users. They have been highly influential in establishing the user movement and in insisting that users have rights. Perhaps their most important contribution has been in demonstrating that what users want and how they perceive their needs can differ in essential aspects from the ways in which professionals and providers define them. User organisations and campaigns have helped to push the agenda for change in the direction of users' interests and towards their participation in service review and development. However, some caution is needed in understanding their viewpoints since several organisations are geared to inform and support the families and relatives of people using residential and other forms of care rather than necessarily serving the interests or protecting the rights of residents themselves.

From our interviews with representatives of user and provider organisations we became aware that there was a great deal of common ground between the care groups and that the distinctions between them might reflect the histories and traditions of service provision rather more than fundamental differences in the needs of the different groups (see Perring 1991).

When we refer to common ground we mean that there was general agreement across the groups, including children and young people. Shared views included:

- that residential care and services would continue to be needed: they were viewed as a kind of facility that could and should be a positive choice. There were many reasons why people saw group care as a benefit: gaining independence from home, moving out of long stay hospital, an opportunity to live with a small group of companions, being looked after in congenial security, breaking with a self-abusive way of life. Negative views expressed related to inadequacies or mismatches in provision or to care approaches rather than residential care in principle;

• there should be a greater voice for people in residential settings, including involvement in planning and decision making. People expected and wanted staff to help them in this but thought many staff would, in turn, need help and support to do so;

• people wanted access to ordinary opportunities for personal development—in day and other activities—through education, social contacts, leisure pursuits and employment;

• and opportunities for self-expression and fulfilment, for friendship and intimate, including sexual, relationships;

• generally people recognised that many limitations in current pro-vision stemmed from inappropriate or outdated models of care. People were advocating a shift from, for example, medical models of treatment to social care based in small group living, ordinary housing and life-styles chosen by the individual;

• users and carers recognised the need for appropriate physical or practical support but they did not necessarily want or expect this to be defined by or met within the home. They wanted to be involved in discussion and to make choices about how such needs might best be met either within or outside an establishment, with or without the support of relatives;

• the issue of being involved in making choices showed that residents did not want their living arrangements—the pattern of their days—to be confined by the home in which they were living;

• there was a universal concern about the viability and financial stability of establishments, about the individual resident's security of tenure and about the security of their financial arrangements.

These concerns in many ways match and mirror the principles for good care provision and practice set out by the *Wagner Review* (Wagner, 1988), by *Home Life* (Centre for Policy in Ageing, 1984) and by *Homes Are for Living In* (DOH/SSI, 1989a).

Residential Care for People from Black and Ethnic Minority Groups

The needs of people from ethnic minorities, elders in particular, are currently poorly addressed in residential care. The two main reasons for this centre on difficulties of access to services and the inappropriateness of the services on offer (SCEMSC, 1986). Both are strongly linked to the prevalence of racist attitudes and institutions which result in discrimination, mistrust and misunderstanding.

The picture from our data base of homes participating in the CHI and from our visits was not encouraging. Generally there were few black residents in homes, even in areas with established ethnic minority communities. There were also few black staff except in areas with high black populations. Black people are generally isolated in residential care, whether workers or residents. The picture varied across care groups, with more black and ethnic minority residents in mental health hostels and in children's establishments.

As a result, black and other groups are increasingly setting up organisations to provide specialist residential care facilities. This is particularly the case for elders who experience particular problems linked to communication and cultural expectations, but also for younger adults with mental health problems who have commonly been offered the more coercive rather than therapeutic forms of service.

The implications for CHI projects were twofold. In order to consider the perspective of black users and potential users, they would have to take a positive and active stance in seeking out establishments catering for black people. They would also need to highlight issues for black and ethnic minority people in all settings, even where these had not been considered.

Care Groups and Their Interests

Although the similarities between care groups seemed to us to outweigh the differences, there are issues about how these more general concerns and principles are translated into arrangements for people living in a particular home. We look now at what was important by using, somewhat reluctantly, the traditional groupings for the moment. The anomalies of trying to arrange services for people who span the care groups—for example, people who are both elderly and mentally ill, youngsters with educational and physical needs, young adults with a learning disability who also need help with a physical difficulty—are frustrating, well known and highlight the need for radical rethinking. But we look briefly at the picture group by group for several reasons:

• policy structures and provider organisations continue to distinguish between people on criteria related to a person's age, physical or mental ability and these will inevitably remain into the foreseeable future;

• equally, professional identity, training, specialisation and career opportunities are strongly determined by care grouping, although this link may be weakened by new community care arrangements;

- many service users draw comfort from a sense of belonging to a group or community of people who are, in important ways, like themselves;

- people do have different needs although these may well relate more to the 'career path' by which people move into and on from residential care than to their age or ability.

The term 'career path' is drawn from Goffman's concept of moral career. It is a way of reflecting the experience of people who enter service institutions (Goffman, 1968). Typically, individuals' needs for support lead them into particular routes and patterns of life. The path which people follow is generally determined by the institutional norms and structures through which services are provided and allocated. These have a profound impact on the life experience of service users.

Therefore, although underlying values and needs are generic, on the whole, care groups do differ in some respects:

- the main reasons for needing residential accommodation or services;

- their pattern of service use: duration of stay, how and when people move out of residential care and the experience of aftercare;

- the prevalent philosophies and types of care offered;

- the strength and stage of development of an organised user voice representing the interests of the care group.

Children and Young People
Children in care include those with special needs due to disability, children who are in care for protection or welfare, due to problems within the family and those with psychological or behavioural problems. A smaller number of children enter residential care through the juvenile justice system, where the object of the service is more overtly one of care with control. The principle of residential care for children and young people as a positive choice, therefore, is complex and subject to continuing debate. The role of parents and attitudes to them will, likewise, be different in each case.

Residential care for children is essentially transitional. For some children it will be short term—a period of assessment and preparation for a fostering or adoption placement—or cyclical, for families who need respite care. For others it is a time of reaching young adulthood and moving towards independence. In all cases, there is a developmental focus as well as provision for the physical and emotional needs of the child.

Young people need to prepare for independence: they have important (and quite ordinary) needs for support on leaving home, yet provision for leaving care is patchy. Removal from previous ties, including kin, friends and schools, make this a particular challenge. Residential establishments should be in a good position to provide continuing and outreach support to young people after leaving but this needs resources and agency support.

Children with disabilities will generally have a continuing need for education, accommodation and care. The transition to adult life is often difficult and usually due to limitations in the services available to support independent living. It is also affected by attitudes of carers and by wider social expectations.

Although voluntary organisations have made an important and often specialised contribution, child care services have been a key responsibility of the statutory sphere. A trend away from long-term residential care towards fostering has resulted in establishments being used increasingly for children with particular problems or for larger sibling groups. For these children, residential care is likely to be a longer term experience and may be in a specialised setting. A scaling down of public provision has led to an unplanned shift towards the private sector which has continued to expand to fill demand for specialised placements from statutory agencies and directly from parents. One result of this is that children can be placed well away from their home area.

The morale of workers in child care has been affected by a series of scandals in the recent past. Successive enquiries have noted lack of training, support and status—problems relevant to all care groups but particularly important for those working with children.

The principle of choice and rights, for children, has tended to be qualified by their minor status, so that it has been difficult for them to articulate their views and have them taken seriously. The Children Act 1989 endorsed the need for children to be involved in decisions about their welfare. Organisations run by children in care, like the National Association of Young People In Care and for children, such as the Voice of the Child in Care, now have a high profile in the media and in policy development and are increasingly invited to comment on child care matters. These have pointed out the possible advantages of good quality residential care, such as peer support and continuity. They have also been active in raising the issues of leaving care and of children's rights while in residential care. However, it is not clear how far this movement has reached large numbers of children in care.

People with Physical Disabilities

This care group includes a wide age range of people with very varied physical or sensory disabilities, requiring different types and levels of support. Many adults with disabilities live in their own homes, either independently or with some degree of support from informal or paid carers. Residential care establishments are often managed by specialist voluntary organisations, catering for particular needs. A number of more 'hotel style' establishments offer holiday or respite care.

The pattern of use of residential care varies according to the nature of the individual's disability and the age at which it developed. Disability needs to be understood as linked to the social and physical environment in which we live: it is often the shortcomings of ordinary facilities which present barriers and may create the need for residential care. However, shifts towards a philosophy of independent living mean that it is increasingly possible for people with quite high levels of need to live in their own accommodation. This means that those who do enter or remain in residential establishments are those with particularly complex needs.

A number of voluntary sector establishments for people with disabilities have a philosophy which regards workers as 'aides'. The aim is for staff to facilitate rather than provide more total care and support. Such philosophies are in contrast to paternalistic forms of care which undermine rather than support independence and personal development. In many care homes, however, it has not been common for residents' views to be given great attention. Most residents are articulate but may need special help to communicate. Many adults with physical disabilities have commented on their frustration with not being listened to seriously.

It is important to recognise that agencies providing specialised facilities for adults with disabilities are not necessarily in a position to speak for them. Equally their families or carers cannot be assumed to have the same interests or perspectives.

Organisations run by people with physical disabilities are emerging and these focus particularly on the wider issues of access, discrimination and stigma which affect all disabled people. User organisations in their campaigns to change attitudes to disability and the role of charity, in particular, have received media attention but they may have had little impact as yet on residential care provision. Despite recent attempts by MPs, there is still no legislation on discrimination against disabled people and some of the key sections of the Disabled Persons Act 1986 have not been implemented. This legislative picture applies to all adults with disabilities, including people with mental health problems.

People with Learning Disabilities
For people with learning disabilities, a move into residential care may be towards greater independence and away from a large scale institution or the parental home. It can, therefore, be understood as a rehabilitative or developmental option. Residents may move in time from more institutional forms of residential care, such as hostels, to more independent forms, such as group homes and supported flats. For many, living and working in ordinary facilities is the aim, but residential care is seen as a positive move towards this.

Services have, until recently, been dominated by medical models of care and by a concern to provide protection or training. However, ideas about quality of care for people with learning disabilities have been influenced, since the 1970s, by principles of normalisation. As a result, residential care is increasingly being provided in smaller units which aim to facilitate greater independence.

Independent user organisations like People First and, most recently Black People First, have been set up and these play a role in encouraging an emphasis on social integration and rights of citizenship. They have focused on the issues of hospital closure, moves towards small group living, education and work opportunities and changing public attitudes. The experience of stigma is still a major concern and they wish to see their lives as valued. It is of key importance, therefore, that residential care should promote participation by individuals in their communities, through education, work, leisure and social ties.

Advocacy schemes and self advocacy are further ways in which people with learning disabilities can have a voice. These developments are of particular importance in demonstrating how, given the right opportunities and support, people can participate and comment on a wide range of matters. Organisations such as People First have also begun to play a role in training practitioners and in service evaluation.

People with Mental Health Problems

The dominance of the medical model of care for people with mental health problems has led to a concentration of resources in the health sector. Voluntary and private provision has increased recently with the movement towards hospital closures but it remains relatively uncommon for people to obtain access to residential care, except through hospital.

The path for most residents is from hospital, on a long-term or repeated pattern of admission, to a period spent in community-based residential care. The aim of hostels and therapeutic communities is generally to prepare people for more independent housing, perhaps in a series of progressive steps. For older residents, who may have lived in an asylum for many years, residential care is more likely to be regarded as permanent, even where there is a focus on rehabilitation.

A particular concern, for people with mental illness, is the way in which the perception of their special needs influences the nature of provision. The principle of choice is often limited because the service user's insight or psychological stability is questioned. User and advocacy organisations which developed through the 1980s underline the validity and practical value of resident participation within homes and within the planning process. These groups are concerned to shift residential care more firmly into the sphere of social care to address what are essentially social needs for a supportive but ordinary home environment. Having gained acceptance of their basic right to consultation, the emphasis now is on effective participation and impact on decisions at all service levels. A large number of local and national user groups exist but these have, so far, failed to gain the kind of public awareness or understanding that, perhaps, other care groups have achieved.

People with Drug or Alcohol Related Problems

The patterns of entry into and use of services, for these groups, are quite different from those commonly associated with residential care. People often experience problems over a number of years and may only seek help reluctantly. The common aim of therapeutic change for the person in residential care involves both intervention and control.

Residential facilities, therefore, generally provide short-term care aimed at altering self-abusive habits and lifestyles. The approach differs according to the therapeutic philosophies of providers, across age groups and between those who have alcohol or drug problems. The former have often lost stable social networks and many become homeless and rootless. Many experience spells in psychiatric hospitals. People with drug problems, on the other hand, are likely to be younger and aiming to return to education or a working life. Service users may experience several periods of residence in facilities of different types before moving on to independent accommodation or achieving personal stability.

Whereas loss of personal ties is generally recognised as a problem of residential care, the aim of residential drug or alcohol services may be to detach people from former networks which encouraged or maintained self-abusive behaviour. Because of the smaller numbers of people involved, and the differences outlined above, facilities are not generally provided on a local basis. The majority of establishments are managed by specialist voluntary organisations and serve regional catchment areas.

Despite the prevalence of therapeutic community approaches, which emphasise communication and collective activity, user groups have not developed strongly. The paradox for people in such facilities is that 'speaking up' is aimed at personal rather than institutional change. As a result, it is still the specialist care group organisations which represent people with drug or alcohol related problems rather than users themselves.

People who are in residential care, across this range of client groups (and also, increasingly people who are homeless and rootless and people with HIV/Aids) share the problem of stigma in some degree. They may be regarded as a threat or simply an embarassment in their neighbourhood. Again, residential care which is isolated has contributed to inaccurate images and assumptions about facilities which are seen as a blight, rather than an integral part of their neighbourhood.

Elders

By referring to elders we imply the respect that some cultures traditionally afford the senior members of their community. We noted, for example, the way Asian elders, however confused, were treated with deference in a home run by an Asian housing association—in contrast to many of the homes for elderly people we visited.

Older people entering residential care will generally do so from their own (family) homes or after a hospital stay. The move may be precipitated by a crisis such as illness or bereavement or by increasing physical or mental frailty. It may take place only when informal carers no longer feel able to cope and so may be accompanied by feelings of loss, guilt or anger. Support for carers, as well as direct services for elders in the community, is an important issue in developing residential and other care services.

Residential care may be rehabilitative (eg. after an illness) but is more commonly viewed as permanent, thereby increasing the feelings of loss on entry into the home. The pervasive tendency to assume that dependency will increase with age discourages homes from considering rehabilitation. So, attempts to improve the quality of life for elders in residential care must address a number of problems at personal and institutional levels.

It is the case that elders suffer forms of stigma experienced to some degree by all care groups and they are often even more isolated from personal or local networks. Organisations of and for elders do not have a high profile amongst those in residential care. Residents' committees, for example, often fulfil a nominal or social function. On the whole, elders are reticent about putting their views forward or making complaints, suggesting that institutionalism is as much a problem for them as for people who have lived in large, long-stay hospitals.

User-oriented organisations, such as Age Concern, Help the Aged, Counsel and Care for the Elderly, are active in providing information and advice for older people and their carers. On the other hand, user-run advice organisations, such as Pensioner's Link, have had little connection with residential care and campaigning has generally taken place at a more national level on issues such as pensions.

Elders with Dementia (Alzheimer's Syndrome)

Homes for elders usually include a number of people experiencing some degree of dementia. There are also specialist homes, with growing provision in the private sector. Residential care for people with dementia must address itself particularly to the need to provide security and to prevent further confusion as a result of the move into care.

There is a widespread assumption that elders with dementia are not able to make positive choices or comment about their situation. It requires time, skill and a positive attitude to enable their views to be expressed. There are, however, an increasing number of encouraging cases where relatives, volunteers and care workers have found ways to assist people with dementia to express their views about their lives in residential care.

Unfortunately, there remains a widespread tendency to view people with dementia as no longer people. Due to their communication and cognitive problems, it has been organisations run for and by their relatives and carers which have been the most involved in representing their needs. However, here, as in all care groups, there are differences between the needs of carers and the needs of residents.

Conclusion

As we have noted, the contexts of residential care and the sets of interests involved, were crucial to the work and the outcomes of the CHI Programmes. The period has been one of intense change. Many people working and living in residential care feel isolated from wider networks and institutions which, nevertheless, impinge on the nature and quality of residential care in a number of ways.

CHI Programmes needed to consider all these spheres of interest in

- planning the scope and balance of project work;

- negotiating involvement, aims and plans with project participants;

- supporting the project work;

- drawing project learning into general guidelines;

- making connections with the structures which would influence the way the work might be implemented, sustained and taken up more widely.

In the chapters to follow, we explore the ways in which each Programme responded to these challenges before going on to look at the meaning and likely outcomes of the work for quality in residential care.

PART TWO

The Development
Programmes

Preamble

THE DEVELOPMENT PROGRAMMES

In the following chapters we describe and comment on the work of each of the research Programmes.

The design of CHI meant that each Programme pursued their research independently with no direct utilisation of the work of others. There were no projects specifically set up to test the links between the Programmes or how far the different approaches could be integrated in practice. A few homes are currently using materials from all Programmes but their experience is not available at the time of writing (Care Weekly, 4.2.93). There were, however, common bases for the work and ones which contributed to some convergence of approach: these we discuss later.

To avoid confusion we refer to the research areas as Programmes and identify each by the letters of the institute or agency responsible. The work on information, for example, we refer to as the PSI Programme, that on training for care staff as the NISW Programme.

General Aspects of the Programmes

Since the four Programmes were based on the recommendations of the Wagner review, the work was founded on similar sets of *values and assumptions* about the nature and purpose of residential care and the principles on which care provision and practice are based.

The Programmes were working to a broadly similar *set of objectives*: to explore and formulate approaches to care practice that would promote the interests of residents and the quality of their life. There were no preconceptions about how the work of the Programmes might be integrated or if the approaches they developed would, when taken up by providers and practitioners, prove compatible.

The general *shape of the work* undertaken, in each case, was also similar. Programmes first defined and shaped the research through reference to current thinking about good practice in their field. The tasks were those of translating principles for practice into plans and working arrangements that were relevant and feasible. Pilot, exploratory and trial projects were set up in collaboration with care establishments and agencies as a means of testing possibilities and learning from the results.

Meetings of the Programme managers with the C & E Group considered aspects of general importance on which the CHI could adopt a common policy.

Coverage of Care Groupings and Sectors

All Programmes intended to include six care groups in their work: children and young people, elders, people with mental health problems, people with learning disabilities, people with physical disability or sensory impairment, and people with drug or alcohol problems.

It was agreed that establishments providing for each of the care groupings should be included in sufficient numbers to ensure that issues of particular importance would be recognised. It was accepted that homes for elders would be the most numerous but not at the expense of other care groups. In the event, the pattern of coverage reflected, rather, the broad distribution of residential provision and fewer establishments for people with drug and alcohol problems, physical disability and children participated than had been hoped (see Appendix 4).

Evaluation Criteria

The key questions which were applied in evaluating the research were:

- how far the work of the Programmes and the approaches they developed were successful in defining and implementing good practice

- how far these helped to promote quality of life.

The Department of Health asked that particular aspects should be considered:

- the value for money they represent

- the level of consumer satisfaction

- their relevance, ease of implementation and transferability.

In addition the C & E Group, together with the Programmes, included equal opportunities and anti-discriminatory service provision as important indicators of good practice and service quality.

A series of internal working papers explored the definition of each of the key evaluative criteria and the general approaches adopted are now outlined.

Value for money

In assessing value for money we were concerned with basic questions about whether an activity was feasible and worthwhile in relation to its costs. In the context of residential care the worth of a project involved a number of perspectives—particularly those of the intended beneficiaries, the residents. This was a qualitative rather than a quantitative assessment. Equally, the notion of cost included quantifiable aspects like staff time, redeployment or staff coverage and financial costs and also qualitative aspects like the degree of effort involved (Brunel/CHI, 1990a). This was an approach which sought to relate the costs in terms of time, effort and money with the value of the outcomes as perceived by staff and, where possible to obtain, residents.

Overall we were interested in the resources and costs necessary to implement the approaches and guidelines finally produced by the Programmes. This meant taking out the extra time and costs involved in the research element of their developments while understanding that implementation might require some form of support from outside the care home. The variety of projects gave an indication of the cost elements involved and, therefore, a guide to the likely resource implications of using the Programmes' final guidelines.

Ease of implementation and transferability

Since the intention was that the materials produced should be relevant across the sectors and care groupings it was important to assess the ease with which they could be implemented or adapted for use in different contexts (Brunel/CHI, 1990b).

In evaluation we looked at the kind of factors which helped or hindered the projects and their effectiveness and how far the Programmes were able to identify and address potential difficulties in the approaches they formulated.

Consumer satisfaction

Consumer satisfaction was taken to refer to the views of the resident or direct service user. Indirect interests were recognised—for example, the relatives, carers and families of residents, the local community and also those of intermediaries—for example, staff, advocates and professionals in other agencies (Brunel/CHI, 1990c). But, for the purposes of evaluating the Programmes' work, residents were taken as the primary consumers: it was their experience, needs, views and wishes which counted in determining levels of satisfaction. Such views were rarely attributable to the project work alone: usually residents were talking more generally about their life and experience in an establishment. But there were cases—especially in the IQA work—where residents were involved in projects and could comment directly.

Black and Ethnic Minority Group Interests and Anti-Discriminatory Practice

The interests of black and ethnic minority groups were not an evaluation theme as such. It was agreed that these should be an essential consideration in all aspects of service provision, review and development and, therefore, in the conduct of all aspects of the research not only in evaluating the Programmes' work. The Programmes adopted a policy and guidelines for anti-discriminatory practice (Brunel/CHI 1990d) which took the view that discrimination is based on perceptions of, and reactions to, difference and, therefore, addressed the interests of all who suffer discrimination on whatever grounds.

The elimination of discrimination, the promotion of equal rights and opportunities for all sections of the community and, in particular, the provision of ethnically sensitive services were seen as essential aspects of good care practice. It was acknowledged that residential care homes provide for a wide range of people whose needs are frequently poorly served and who have been passively or actively discriminated against because of their age, disability, gender, state of health (e.g. HIV/Aids, epilepsy), sexuality, race, colour, religion or social class.

An annotated bibliography on black perspectives was produced to help identify issues for practice, service review and development (Youll & Aindow 1991).

Describing the Programmes of Research

The following chapters describe and comment on each Programme. They are organised according to a systems approach which looks at the relationship between inputs, the processes, outputs and outcomes of the developmental work.

Inputs: the thinking and planning that shaped the projects and the resources to run them, came from the researchers at Programme level and from the managers and staff of the participating homes. The work undertaken in all the projects was the result of negotiation between the Programme and local interests.

Processes: the means by which the projects were set up and run varied considerably across CHI but all involved the co-operation of a number of different people. The relationships, interactions and arrangements between them were an important part of the learning of the projects and were an essential element in demonstrating how change might be initiated and implemented.

Intermediate outcomes: each project had its own terms of reference, specific objectives and intended outcomes. Each could, therefore, be assessed as to how far these aims had been achieved. But in terms of the Programme and CHI as a whole, these were intermediate outcomes, i.e., the results that helped to shape the Programmes' final products. We discuss these as they relate to residents, staff and others involved in the care establishments. The outcomes of the project were useful indicators of the results which might be expected from using the Programmes' final publications and materials.

Outputs: the published materials that resulted from the work both project (local) and Programme (generic) levels.

Final outcomes: the final results of the work can only be assessed as others put to use the approaches which the Programmes developed. The answer to questions about how far the work will help to ensure quality of life for residents will be answered when a sufficient number of homes and agencies have had the opportunity to use and comment on the guidelines and other materials produced by the Initiative.

Chapter 3

INSIDE QUALITY ASSURANCE: INTERNAL REVIEW FOR RESIDENTIAL HOMES

Two key aspects which the Wagner review highlighted were the importance of independent inspection and service review. It advocated that all establishments should be subject to the same system but did not consider this would be sufficient to set and maintain high standards: periodic in-house review was also required.

The review made clear recommendations that residential care providers

'should promote systems of self-evaluation and performance review ... no new establishment should be registered which is not prepared to adopt such a system.' (p59) and that these should include, 'the expressed wishes and views of residents and their relatives' as well as staff at all levels' (p57).

(Wagner, 1988)

The Centre for Environmental and Social Studies in Ageing (CESSA) at the Polytechnic of North London (now University of North London) was commissioned to develop a system of in-house self assessment and performance review. The aim was to develop a package flexible enough to work in different types of care homes, involving staff, residents and outsiders and accessible enough to enable home managers and proprietors to run the review themselves.

The Programme team adopted the title 'Inside Quality Assurance' (IQA) to reflect the internal nature of the review and to convey a more accessible and friendly view of the task.

Inside   – the home itself conducts the review
Quality   – the key focus of the review
Assurance   – a positive approach.

The Challenge

There were several challenges to the development of any system of internal review but especially a system involving residents and care workers at all levels.

First, the studies of the CESSA team (Willcocks et al, 1987; Peace et al, 1982; Weaver et al, 1985) and those working on the development of complaints procedures show how reticent direct service users are in commenting on their experience. The reasons for this are well known: people do not want to risk upsetting those on whom they depend for their care and security. There was plenty of evidence from our visits to establishments and talks with residents, their relatives and with care staff that this caution, justified or not, is the norm. How then to ensure that residents not only have the opportunity to comment but also feel safe to do so? The Programme also needed to consider how to enable people with sensory impairment, communication or learning disabilities to participate fully.

Second, care staff are no more likely than residents to be confident about commenting on current practice and standards in a home. There have been a disquieting number of instances where staff who have attempted to question care practice or 'blow the whistle' have been ignored or effectively silenced by senior management (Kelly, 1993). The setting up of a support group *Freedom to Care* for people who speak out about bad practice testifies to the difficulties and fears of staff in medical, nursing and legal practice. There is no widely established tradition of seeking the views of frontline workers in social care services and the generally low status and morale of residential workers means that they are even less likely to give their views freely. How might a system ensure that frontline staff too are able to contribute to internal review?

Third, the system would have to address the issue of how to deal with individual views, whether from resident, staff or relative. If a review is to involve all those with an interest in the home, then all contributions have to be taken seriously. In group living situations the difficulty of reconciling idiosyncratic, individual views and preferences with the needs of the collective are well known. How to set up a way of obtaining views which does not lead to false expectations or misrepresentation?

Fourth, the researchers were well aware that homes are run by people with their own interests and needs. For owner-managers the home is their livelihood; for care managers and staff the home is their workplace and they too have rights as people and as employees. They are people who have built up experience and knowledge over the years and are strongly identified with the work they do. Their views on the running of the home may not entirely coincide with those of the residents. How may a system of review lead to a reasonable balance between different ideas and interests?

Fifth, there were issues to be taken into account about the value or otherwise of linkage between an internal system of review and the quality assurance and inspection procedures which are originated outside the home by the encompassing agency or by independent inspection units. How far should the internal process be shaped or influenced by external norms and criteria?

How the Work was Developed

Value bases and overall approach
The guiding principle of the research was the centrality of the residents' experience. It is the quality of their life which is of prime importance and

their understanding should be central in defining, assessing and reviewing quality. Traditionally, the power to shape services comes from those at the top, even though they are the most distant from the everyday experience of the service. The IQA model starts with those at the core of residential life—residents and frontline staff.

The researchers drew on their previous research and experience in residential care for the elderly. The key feature of this was the assumption that residential establishments involve a number of different groups of people. One of the tasks of review would be to look at the balance or possible tensions between residents' interests and staff interests, even though staff view themselves as working for the benefit of residents. Earlier work had shown that organisational interests often prevail.

There were also potential tensions between the interests of individuals and the residential group as a whole. Whereas in other institutional settings—such as workplace, school or day services—such conflicts of interest may occupy only a part of people's time and experience, for people in full-time residential care such problems can dominate their lives. The families and carers of people in care establishments also have needs and rights and their interests, too, enter into the balance.

The work of the CESSA team was, therefore, based on understanding the care home as involving the concerns and interests of insiders and outsiders. The basic value position was that review should involve all those with an interest in the home but that the needs and views of residents should take primacy. It is important to note that the work was based on obtaining the views of individuals and, as such, was qualitative. The researchers were interested in enabling people to comment as individuals rather than in drawing up or defining generic standards.

The Programme team made an early decision to develop one model of internal review but one which described an accessible and adaptable process. It was to address the practical issues of *how to* run a review as well as describe *what* should be done in the interests of good practice.

Phases of the work
The work was developed in three phases, included all care groups and sectors, and involved the participation of 109 establishments in all (see Appendix 4.4.2).

Pilot work
The pilot projects drew on the researchers' experience of residential care for elders. This knowledge was used to draw up a set of topics for a draft questionnaire which was piloted with residents, care workers and others in a home for children and young people, one for elders and one for physically disabled people.

Developmental stage
At this stage the interview schedule was refined and an overall process and structure was developed. The researchers took the lead in conducting

interviews, steering the process and writing up a report. They were thus action researchers in the full sense: learning first hand what worked in practice, recording and analysing their experience. They functioned both as outsiders and (inevitably) as assumed experts. They were a considerable resource to the homes at this stage, in initiating the review and carrying it through.

Trial round
Building on the development phase, a system was designed and published as a prototype manual and set of materials. This was tried by over 100 homes without support from the Programme. The aims were to see if the materials were sufficient to enable people to run a review and to use their feedback to make final revisions to the IQA system. Participants were asked to comment on their progress and give their views by completing two short questionnaires mid-way through and at the end of the process.

Those participating ranged across sectors of provision, client groups and regions and included a wide range of establishment types and sizes. They were recruited through letters to social service managers and inspectors, care associations and general CHI publicity. The researchers did not rely on existing networks or contacts at this stage: many of the participants knew little about quality assurance models or what the IQA pack would be like.

A significant number of home managers found themselves 'volunteered' by enthusiastic line managers or owners. A number of homes from one agency took part, but these were not, on the whole, managed as organised groups. A few voluntary organisations viewed the exercise as a trial run for the agency and selected a range of homes accordingly.

An orientation meeting was held for those interested in participating and was followed by a series of regional meetings for homes running trials. Otherwise there was no support for the work.

Learning from each stage was systematically fed into the next phase, allowing progressive pulling together, refinement and testing. The IQA system, therefore, draws strongly on the experience of the Programme team, practical advice and feedback from agency and line managers, home managers and staff, residents, carers and other people concerned with the quality of residential care.

The IQA system
The central feature of the system is the Quality Group. This is convened to run the review and is distinct from the formal lines of management and day-to-day running of the home.

The IQA pack (CESSA, 1992) contains a detailed step-by-step description of the process and a set of basic tools. People using the system are encouraged to adapt these materials to suit their specific needs or to create new ones where necessary.

Value base

The IQA system is based in a coherent set of values. These are made explicit but are also implicit in the methods chosen.

> 'Adopting the IQA approach means that the residents are seen as the key evaluators. The message comes through loud and clear that residents' wishes and concerns about living in the home are respected. Staff and others who know the home are also asked what they think, but, from the residents' "perspective".' (PNL/CESSA, 1992)

The process takes account of principles and current thinking about good practice which are reflected in the structure and processes described in the pack. Emphasis is placed on helping people to have a say and on listening. Throughout, attention is drawn to the values underpinning the exercise—people are prompted to think about the reason for the review and to focus on residents' quality of life.

Stages

The first step in the process is to clarify the *purposes and objectives* of the home as an important basis for setting clear standards and expectations. Like the NISW work on training the materials emphasise the benefit of staff, managers and residents having a shared view of what the home is providing or seeking to achieve.

The hub of the review is the *Quality Group*. The manual specifically advises that representatives of residents, staff, relatives and other outside interests constitute the group and that the care home manager or proprietor is neither a member nor takes the chair. The aim is to convene a group that is able to operate in a relatively independent way while utilising both the direct knowledge and experience of insiders balanced with the more distanced interest of outsiders.

The task of the Quality Group is to obtain, collate and write up a report on the views and comments of residents and staff and where possible relatives.

Outsider members of the Quality Group *interview residents and staff.* The interview questionnaires are based on seven topics: physical care; making choices; expressing feelings; the home as somewhere to live; knowing how things run; making links; how the home feels to residents. Two simple questions are asked of each: what is it like here? and what needs to be different? There are more detailed prompts but, again, the questions are designed to be unthreatening, colloquial and open ended enough to allow people to respond with their own preoccupations and priorities. The Quality Group is encouraged to revise or add topics and questions to ensure that they are relevant to the home and its residents.

Confidentiality is an issue and the pack alerts the quality group to address this. If it is important that individuals are not identified, the quality group has a responsibility to ensure that this is respected. The pack provides guidance on the purposes of interviewing and how best to approach residents and others. Again the emphasis is on helping people to speak out. Some attention is given to possible ways of creating opportunities for people with sensory or speech impairment, like using prompt cards or the services of an advocate. The pack includes, for example, an extract describing a technique for use with people with cognitive impairment as a way of 'breaking the silence' (Iveson, 1990).

IQA advises that the responses are looked at as a collection rather than a series of individual commentaries. This helps to discourage undue emphasis on the responses of individuals and encourage an understanding of the general messages coming through. Clusters of concern, the general tenor of the comments and any mismatches between what people are saying and the values of the home can be noted by the Quality Group.

The comments are collated and fed back to residents and to staff as a means of *checking* that the Group's understanding of the issues raised is sufficiently accurate. This is one way in which different views can be recognised and the balance between idiosyncratic and more collective views can be discussed.

The review is then written up in *a report* which gives an account of the results, identifies issues and forms the basis of decision making and action. The pack encourages the Quality Group to plan for the next IQA review and to think about using the document to inform people about the home.

Learning from the IQA Trials

Drawing on our own fieldwork we now discuss some of the main comments and observations from the homes and agencies which tried out the IQA materials. We were also able to analyse responses received from participant homes by the CESSA team, from home managers and Quality Group Chairs. Of ninety-seven homes surveyed, forty-seven responses were received of which fifteen were also studied in our field visits. We concentrate here on the practicalities and experience of running an in-house review: in the next section we focus on the results of the process for residents, staff and the home as a whole.

Using the Pack

The evidence from the trials suggests that home care managers and those involved in quality groups found the pack comprehensive, informative and user friendly. The materials, although detailed and quite lengthy, led people through the process in a logical way and, as far as we know, none of the few homes to drop out did so because they could not follow the process. Generally people were positive about the presentation, layout and general approach. Many quality groups had successfully undertaken revisions to make the system more relevant. We were interested to note that homes working independently in the trial round were more confident in making changes and adapting the IQA materials than those involved in earlier phases which were supported by a CESSA researcher.

A few managers had expected the exercise to be very structured and to focus on defining and measuring quality standards. Most, however, compared the qualitative approach favourably with more statistical and structured approaches to review—like the use of checklists or standard indicators.

Above all, the pack provided the information and guidance necessary for homes to set up and run a review independently. Some home managers were able to discuss progress with others in their agency or consult with a senior manager but, on the whole, people managed by using the pack itself and making their own decisions about how to proceed.

Motivations for Participating

When asked about their reasons for taking part, most managers spoke of their interest in reviewing and improving quality. A number expected that some system of quality assurance would be required under contracting arrangements and wanted to get ahead by developing their own expertise. Managers were also interested in trying new ideas and keeping up with quality initiatives.

Interest in, and awareness of, quality assurance grew rapidly during the life of the Programme and a number of managers were responding to this general trend. A few stated their motives as being basically 'cynical'—that is, concerned with the reputation of the establishment, but then went on to talk about a range of other possible benefits, including hearing residents' views.

A number of managers wanted to promote the involvement of residents and saw IQA as a way of empowering which was more than establishing a resident-centred view of quality. The involvement of outsiders, including people in the local community, was welcomed together with opportunities for staff to give their views. Although few residents were involved in the decision to conduct a review, most saw it as a worthwhile opportunity to comment.

Quality Groups and Their Membership

The Quality Group comprised insiders (people who live and work in the home) and outsiders (people with an interest in the home) reflecting a balance of interests, including residents, care staff, people in senior positions, relatives and so on. This balance was not always achieved in practice. Ideas about who was an outsider varied greatly: some establishments only involved other professionals or people with a working relationship to the home and its residents; others were determined to include people who were completely independent from the establishment and its managing agency. Similarly, while some groups were chaired by home managers, others felt strongly that they should not take a dominant, or even active, part in the process.

The role of the Quality Group Chair

The role of the Chair was crucial in two ways. First, the Quality Group had to be convened, and to develop a sense of purpose and clarity about the tasks to be undertaken. This leadership position was not always easy for outsiders to take on and this related to the second aspect of the role. The Quality Group is set up as a semi-independent forum through which a review can be conducted. As such it stands alongside but, in important respects, separate from day-to-day management. Many homes found that sorting out the relationship between Chair and home manager was crucial. Some avoided the issue because the home manager chaired the Quality Group but there was a general recognition of the possible tension between the two roles.

Resident involvement in Quality Groups

Participation by residents in Quality Groups was generally low but the reasons for this were instructive. In most cases it was the manager who decided which residents to approach based on who they felt would be able and willing. Relatively little use was made of residents' groups or committees to decide who should represent them on the group. Few homes had experience of involving residents in any kind of formal meeting and had not realised that residents might need help if they were to participate. For example, two elderly residents found it difficult to get involved in one group because there was a general lack of explanation from the home manager or Chair of the group. In contrast, another chairperson took time to prepare the room and to introduce the meeting in a helpful way after residents experienced problems in the first meeting. As a result they were able to take a more active part. In another home, two elderly residents attended but remained unclear about their role: one commented 'We had tea and sandwiches and they talked amongst themselves.'

Staff in some homes assumed that residents would not want or be able to participate in this way. For example, a view held in one home was that the residents—young adults with learning disabilities—were too prone to mood swings for their views to be useful. Elsewhere staff expressed strong doubts that elderly people 'wanted to be bothered' with interviews or that they might be upset by the experience.

Where residents were active on the quality group, the outcomes of the review showed that their contribution had been significant. Only a few homes used advocates as a means of helping residents although one or two invited members of user or advocacy organisations to join in the Group themselves. A few homes invited former residents to join the Quality Group and found their contribution very helpful, especially in interviewing both residents and staff.

An underlying problem, then, was the attitude of staff towards the residents and the assumptions made about their capacity to comment. Even where their right to participate was accepted, many residents were effectively prevented from speaking out.

Staff involvement in Quality Groups

Nearly all Quality Groups included staff and efforts were generally made to ensure that basic level workers and domestic staff were represented. Several appointed junior staff to chair the group and this produced interesting anomalies of responsibility and in leadership, particularly where the home manager was also a member. Groups struggled with getting a balance between staff and residents, between different staff grades and length of service. It was interesting that people did not give up in the face of difficulties of this sort and this may reflect a hope that the insider-outsider balance might help contain, moderate or find solutions to such issues. In a sense, these efforts highlighted the issues of power and interest that underlie everyday life and work. Staff members were often puzzled about how to carry out their role on the group—should they speak for themselves?—for their colleagues?—for 'their' residents?

Involvement of outsiders in Quality Groups

Participation by relatives appeared to depend mainly on the nature of residents' family relationships and, again, it was managers who tended to take the lead in deciding who to contact. In some settings family links were not strong, while in others, the involvement of relatives was seen as a potential problem. Establishments for young adults, for example, viewed residents as independent people whose relatives should have no special voice or influence. Establishments for children on the other hand (despite agreement in principle) were anxious about involving parents in practice.

In most cases, outsiders on the quality group took an active, even leading, role in carrying out the review, from planning and interviewing to sorting the information and writing the report. In nearly all cases, it was very much a collaborative exercise. This was encouraging since, in earlier phases, home managers had found difficulty in involving outsiders or ensuring that they took an active role.

Our interviews suggested that a great deal of effort and thought went into finding Quality Group members. Many managers commented that it was difficult to find and recruit people with the time and energy to commit to the work.

Lay outsiders on Quality Groups included priests, relatives, JPs, existing volunteers, former residents, members of Leagues of Friends and members of local community organisations. People who were outsiders, but had some professional interest in the home included GPs, community nurses, therapists, social workers, social work students on placement, probation officers, teachers, managers or workers from other residential homes or day services.

Difficulty in recruiting outsiders prompted homes into more creative thinking about who might be approached and some of the most productive links came from involving former residents. Many involved people who had a more direct interest in the home, such as inspectors and agency training officers. In these cases their involvement was regarded as beneficial for other purposes, such as the development of quality approaches in the wider agency.

There were also homes where a line manager was seen as an outsider because they did not actually work within the home. But there were always conflicts here as to who was competent to guide decisions and take action: internal or external management?

Interviewing

The purpose of the interviews was to provide an opportunity for people to comment freely as individuals. The pack advises that interviewing should be done by outsiders on the Quality Group.

Residents speak out

Nearly all homes in the trial round were successful in interviewing most of their residents. A number of residents said that they did not mind being interviewed but stressed that they did not wish to complain. It was notable that a number of residents were so unfamiliar with being asked their views, they felt it would imply complaining or fussing in some way to comment at all. Other residents took a more positive view, describing the interviews as interesting and enjoyable and a good idea. A number said that, although they had no problems themselves, they felt the exercise would be very important for residents who did. Residents in one home stressed to us that their comments were mainly positive, but they still felt it was right they should be asked their views: the fact of being asked was a positive feature of the home and they compared their situation favourably with that of other people who, they knew, were less happy and did not have the chance to talk about how they felt.

On the whole, residents confirmed that it was better to be interviewed by outsiders—it helped people to speak freely or critically—but a known and trusted outsider was better than a complete stranger. In a home for people with learning disabilities staff felt ambivalent about the use of outsiders because of their limited communication skills: some residents had been anxious and had needed more time to feel comfortable with the interviewer. Several staff feared residents would associate the review with change and be worried about the motives behind it. An elderly resident told us she had agreed to be interviewed but she did not complain because she was 'happy living in the home and did not wish to move'. Such comments highlight the underlying anxieties that so many residents experience about security and acceptance.

Few residents declined the opportunity to be interviewed. There were two cases reported of interviews not completed because the resident had become distressed. On the other hand, staff in one home noticed how an elderly woman with dementia was more alert and communicative after the interview. In two homes, staff expressed some doubts about whether interviewing, in the usual sense, was the best approach for people with learning and communication difficulties. Nonetheless, they felt the process could be improved with experience and saw the overall exercise as worthwhile. In one home, staff were surprised by how many residents had been able to respond.

The practical issues of creating opportunities for people with sensory, cognitive or speech impairment were tackled by a number of homes. Some found the prompt cards in the IQA pack useful, some used advocates, others tried a group discussion approach, others asked relatives or friends to help. Although this aspect of IQA practice was not strongly developed, the experience of the trial homes suggested that no care group should be considered too problematic to contribute to a review.

For many residents, therefore, being asked to comment was a new experience, but one that was positive and worthwhile. Residents them-selves saw a value in being involved in thinking and talking about their own situation and the home as a whole. Although not all were sure that the approach would deal with serious problems they considered that IQA was a step in the right direction.

Care staff speak out

The response of care staff varied widely. In a number of establishments, the review was initially greeted with suspicion and some resistance. This was more likely, unsurprisingly, where staff were not well consulted or prepared or were not actively involved except through the interviews. Some staff initially declined interviews but expressed interest later when they heard from colleagues. Initial anxiety about the nature or purpose of the review was common but this generally declined once the process was under way and better understood.

On the whole, staff said they enjoyed the interviews and found them interesting. Staff were asked to comment from the residents' point of view and Quality Group interviewers were unsure about how to interpret staff comments. Some felt this was ambiguous or difficult for staff to do. Some care staff pointed out that the residents are really the only people who can give their view and suggested it would more more informative if staff gave their own views. Staff in one home felt quite strongly that IQA interviews should focus on staff needs; they saw a direct connection between meeting staff needs—such as for better training—quality of staff practice and quality of care for residents.

The response of both residents and care staff to the exercise may have been affected by the way it was explained and introduced. The general pattern was that this was not handled very well and so it is encouraging that most residents and staff responded positively. In most cases it was the home manager alone who decided to participate in the trial and other staff or residents were only consulted later. The level of explanation offered varied greatly but the main effort had gone into recruiting quality group members. As a result, not all staff understood clearly the purpose or nature of the review although many came to do so through experience.

Making Sense of the Information

There were two main issues about analysing the information gathered from the interviews: handling the volume and interpreting the comments.

Analysing the volume of information from interviews represented a considerable challenge for establishments, particularly those with large numbers of residents and staff and those not accustomed to written procedures. The prototype pack was seen as helpful in giving clear guidance on this part of the exercise. In most cases it was felt appropriate that this should be led by the outsiders. Although the degree of sophistication of presentation varied, all the groups which completed interviews managed the analysis, with much work being done by Quality Group Chairs or home managers.

Feedback meetings with staff and with residents were valued as a way of checking interpretations and impressions and were important in producing more responses from residents and staff. Several managers mentioned how these discussions had led to a revival or creation of a residents' group of some sort.

A key challenge for the Quality Group was in knowing how to interpret the more indirect hints about a problem or a desire for change. Some managers were aware, for example, that a stress on positive comments might reflect residents' caution about airing their views or seeming ungrateful for the genuine care of staff. Comments were often couched within descriptions, rather than given as direct opinions: criticisms were implied behind qualified praise.

Residents also offered comments without indicating what changes they would like to see. Interestingly, staff in a number of homes were more critical, or oriented towards change, than the residents.

One of the underlying problems, anticipated by the researchers, was that the interviews would reveal differences of viewpoint. In a number of cases, staff and residents stressed different things. Although outside participation is important, some quality group members—especially relatives—found it difficult to take a critical approach. One report, for example, provided explanations or rationalisations for critical comments made by residents. One member, the parent of a young adult with learning disabilities, emphasised that parents were not likely to be critical for various reasons: for example, if their son or daughter had moved from a hospital or larger institution and the home compared very favourably. Their expectations, through bitter experience, were fairly low and they were glad to have obtained a place in a long-term residential establishment which was good enough.

The IQA Report, Planning and Action

The final stage of the process was to write up and circulate a report and plan action. Reports were generally drafted by the Quality Group, and then circulated for checking and wider impressions. Given that many establishments had not completed final reports when interviewed, it was useful to note that reports were being used actively in the establishments for discussion and future planning. In many cases, recommendations for change were relatively minor and could be managed within everyday work planning, in staff and resident meetings. A number of homes planned internal work, particularly through staff training, to respond to some of the issues raised. Generally, the reports provided grounded and resident-centred points for action or development.

Some homes developed larger-scale plans, with financial implications, which required approval from senior management. In some cases, these ideas were not entirely new, but the review had shaped up or confirmed existing ideas or shown staff that residents would support their ideas. In one large mental health establishment, for example, staff put in an application for major funding to 'unitise' the building, with a number of long-term implications for the way the hostel would be run. They had already considered the idea, but residents' requests for more choice and individual attention persuaded them to act on the idea. They planned another IQA review once the changes had been made, in order to see what residents felt about the new set-up.

Establishments differed greatly in their intentions about circulating reports: some intended to make it widely available—to show what they had done and be open about their strengths and weaknesses—while others wished to treat it as an internal document. All reports retained anonymity to the degree that names of people were not used, but most were happy to attach the name of the establishment and discuss wider distribution. Some establishments wanted to see the report circulated within their local authority as a way of demonstrating their approach to quality assurance and to quality per se. Once produced, most agreed fully open access within the home and also chose to circulate it within their agency and the local authority. Where initial views had been cautious, follow-up interviews showed greater enthusiasm for using the report and some frustrations about lack of response from their agencies.

The forty-seven homes which provided feedback to CESSA all wished to repeat the exercise. Most considered the review should be a continuous process and probably repeated every one or two years, allowing time for action and follow up in between. A smaller number said they would repeat the exercise with some modifications: suggestions included changes in composition of the Quality Group, involving residents more actively and some minor changes to interview topics or wording of questions. A number of homes saw the initial report as a sort of baseline for comparison with the findings of future reviews. They felt it would make more sense as a comparative exercise over time. A few said they would probably repeat the exercise only when problems or changes in the establishment suggested a need to do so.

Approaches to confidentiality
In developing the pack the Programme team were concerned that, particularly in small settings, confidentiality would be difficult to guarantee and could lead to concern with 'who said what' rather than how to respond to 'what was said' . However, they were also aware that many residents, elders in particular, made very guarded comments and were reluctant to make criticisms.

In interviews with residents and staff, confidentiality was often mentioned and was valued greatly in most cases. A number of residents pointed out that, although they were happy and felt free to say what they thought, they could imagine situations where confidentiality would be crucial to the effectiveness of the exercise.

Care staff valued confidentiality equally highly. Most Quality Groups followed the recommendation to use outsiders as interviewers and felt this made it easier for staff and residents to give their views and a lot of attention was given to matching interviewers and interviewees sensitively. The main exception to this view was where residents had particular communication problems and/or might be worried by an interview with a stranger. In several homes for people with learning disabilities, the resolution was to use a worker who already knew the residents but was not directly connected with staffing of the home. In most cases, outsiders on the Quality Group were known to residents and staff in some way e.g. a local priest or a regular volunteer.

What was Involved in Running an IQA Review?

Duration of the review and effort involved
At the development stage, Programme consultants aimed to work in homes for up to six months. They felt that the review would need to be completed by most homes within about a four-month period for it to be acceptable to managers and to be repeated at regular intervals. In the trial round, the duration of projects was similar—with a period of four to six months being about average. Some variation was explained by the time taken in starting up the process: understanding the pack, explaining the process to others and recruiting Quality Group members. This suggests that, for many homes, a subsequent review could be completed in about three to four months.

A further cause of delay was in writing up the review and this often reflected a lack of confidence in producing formal reports. Many homes had developed plans and begun to take action before a final report was produced and there seemed to be a general reluctance to move from draft to final report. Homes attached importance to the report and the image of the establishment it would portray to a wider interest group.

Most establishments aimed for quite a strict timetable and a first review to take about six months. Considering the pack and organising a quality group took most homes at least a month. It seems reasonable to assume that such work would be easier a second time around, particularly where original Quality Group members continue to take part. On the whole, quality groups did not include people experienced in research, interviewing, analysing written information and so on.

In commenting on the pack, many managers and other participants had initially viewed it as rather daunting and likely to take a great deal of work. These views changed once participants had time to study the manual and get started. At later stages, the general view was that the exercise did take time—some leeway was vital—but it was manageable.

Costs and value for money

The costs of the exercise were not a problem in most cases. The major cost was in the time committed by home managers but many were able to fit the work into ordinary routines. Others pointed out that, however time consuming, it should be seen as part of the home's task and not as an extra cost. Nonetheless, for many homes it was a challenge to find time to carry out the review at a reasonable pace and they relied strongly on the contribution of outsiders. People with such time and commitment were not always easy to find and effort had to go into finding suitable volunteers.

A typical pattern of time costs is outlined below:

• For Quality Group members—eight hours of meetings;

• For interviewers—one hour per interview including preparation plus time to collate the responses;

• For managers—time studying, explaining and introducing IQA to potential Quality Group members, staff and residents and then following up results and taking action through usual management procedures and meetings;

• For Quality Group chairpeople—varying times spent drafting and preparing the report;

• For staff and residents—one hour interview plus feedback and discussion time

Other costs included photocopying of interview sheets and agendas, printing the report and travel allowances for Quality Group members. To this would need to be added the cost of buying the pack for establishments starting in the future. The cost of the pack was regarded as reasonable and compared well with training packs, but many homes do not have budgets for this sort of work.

The Results of Using IQA

We draw here on the feedback obtained by CESSA from the homes which used the prototype pack in the trial round and our own fieldwork. We comment on the results and what they indicate about the kind of outcomes that might be expected from using the final version.

Outcomes for Residents

The outcomes of IQA reviews for residents were considerable in many cases and can be divided into various types.

First was the direct impact on the residents themselves of *being involved* in the process and the review. There were indications that this could be the most significant outcome of an in-house review. Their expectations of the home and of themselves as people able to comment and to be taken seriously were changed considerably in many cases. Even where residents did not say much or speak freely, it seemed that the experience opened up possibilities for the future.

Second was the impact on the *material environment* and running of the home itself, which may have indirect or direct effects on residents' quality of life. Most homes undertook changes in the physical environment or daily routines to meet residents' wishes and ideas.

Third was the impact on the *attitudes and practices* of staff and others, such as outside professionals, relatives and local people. Again, these were expected to have some impact on the quality of residents' lives.

Feedback showed that the majority reported positive developments. All those who returned questionnaires felt there had been some impact: a smaller number suggested quite a high level of impact on the home overall and/or on residents.

A significant number of homes made specific mention of benefits to residents. These included comments that residents were empowered or that they were now being heard more; that residents were involved more and benefited from this; that staff now knew more about residents' needs and wishes. Most had found residents' responses encouraging. The majority felt that IQA would help residents to express their ideas but that the review, on its own, was not sufficient—the work needed reinforcement and support.

Our interviews with residents, staff and Quality Group members suggested that the benefits for residents were strongly related to the manner in which the review was carried out. Where resident involvement was minimal, impact tended to be relatively minor.

It was clear that doing the review in itself had important effects which could become self sustaining. In several homes residents and staff had discovered things about themselves and what they could achieve, as individuals and collectively. Residents gained confidence both in their ability to speak out and in the results of doing so: as positive things began to happen, so it was possible to take things further. In one home, for example, the residents' committee which had previously (according to the manager) been moribund took on a new life and began to pursue issues which had emerged during the review. An interesting incident from one of the demonstration homes was that an elderly resident complained about a member of staff well after the review had ended. It appeared that she had taken time to consider if it was worth complaining and had then chosen when and to whom she would talk.

In contrast, changes achieved by some homes were relatively minor and unlikely to alter the nature of residents' experience to any great extent. In some contexts this was because the residents felt the home was basically good. Children in one home, for example, described a regime which they felt was firm but fair, understandable and helpful to them in various ways. Any changes they wanted were relatively small, such as being able to choose to bath less often. They valued other things, like the attention keyworkers gave to education, checking on homework and so on.

In this and other homes, residents also mentioned issues which the establishment had no power to change—such as the levels of benefits and allowances available. Such issues were important to people's quality of life in residential care, but depended on structures and policies beyond the power of the home or its managing agency to change.

The IQA exercise revealed that residents generally tend to have limited expectations of the home and what can change. Their sights are lowered not only by previous experience—perhaps long-term hospital care—but also by the level of stimulation or challenge in the home itself. Apathy and lack of confidence can quickly set in.

A very small number of homes treated the exercise in a nominal manner, particularly regarding resident and outsider involvement. Consequently, the experience of the review was less challenging than it might have been and made less impact on residents' lives. There is a danger that some homes will focus attention on relatively minor issues, or those thought important by staff while issues of concern to residents are not fully addressed. Even so, there are hints that the expression of views required by the activities may have positive effects in the longer term.

A number of residents whom we interviewed were well aware of the limits of what could be changed through an in-house review. Residents discussed changing the use of the home in radical ways, but were confronted with basic problems in the nature of residential care. Many were sceptical that the review could touch on the underlying problems they experienced of isolation and misunderstanding from the wider society. Nonetheless, it may be significant that they were voicing these issues—perhaps for the first time.

Residents' committees
One area in which changes might become self sustaining was in the effect of the exercise on residents' committees. An increasing number of establishments have such groups but they are often admitted to be ineffective and to involve a minority of residents. Residents' committees often had no proper structure or recognition and no rights or obligations. IQA led to change in the nature and function of some groups, through giving them a greater sense of purpose and increasing resident (and staff) interest. A few groups were actually sparked off by feedback sessions, so that residents themselves began to take issues raised in interviews further.

Residents commented that individual interviews complement committees or other meetings. They allowed quieter people to have a voice and the privacy and confidentiality of the interviews was seen as important. Residents in one home felt that more had happened as a result of the review than their committee had ever achieved. This process was aided by a growth in the confidence of the residents involved: the home's line manager suggested that a year ago, the residents would not have felt confident enough to meet with us for our evaluation.

Relevance for different care groups
The trial of the IQA pack revealed no major difficulties in principle in using the general approach and procedures across the care groups. The significant differences related to the ways in which and the extent to which residents required preparation and help to be a member of a Quality Group and to use the opportunity provided by the interview. The main issues concerned whether staff viewed the resident as able and willing to be interviewed. Young people, people with mental confusion, with communication needs or who displayed emotional instability, were highly likely to be assumed to be unable to comment. A crucial issue is, therefore, to ensure that residents' right to speak out is not subtly eroded by uncritical assumptions about their capacity to do so.

Specific points, we suggest, are the need to clarify the rights and role of the parent in relation to establishments for children and young people and for young adults with learning disabilities, and the need for careful attention to the communication needs of people with sensory or cognitive impairment.

None of the homes involved in the projects specialised in services for ethnic minority communities. Where no or few of current residents are black, issues of particular concern for ethnic minorities may not be highlighted, even though they may form unintentional barriers to people in those communities. How, for example, will a home for elders with all white residents raise the issues of culturally appropriate choices and facilities for other people. One project, a home with all white residents, involved a representative from a local Asian association in the quality group. This member interviewed a number of elderly residents, got to know the home and was then interviewed, along with other members, as part of the evaluation. She was able to provide insight into how the topics covered might have mattered to an elderly person from an ethnic minority. This work helped to raise a number of issues for the home.

A mental health agency was hoping to get the pack translated so they could try it in their hostel for Asian men. The researchers hoped that the topic area on making links would provide an opening to consider the needs and interests of residents from different cultures, backgrounds, racial and cultural communities.

Outcomes for Staff

Staff were involved through the interviews conducted by the Quality Group in which they were asked to think about life from the resident's point of view. This caused some confusion. Many commented that they appreciated the importance of the residents' interests but wanted to comment from their experience as staff—and this is what many did.

Feedback from the Quality Group was, perhaps, the most significant part of the review in terms of influencing staff views and raising awareness of the ideas, needs and perceptions of others. There was evidence that many staff groups were able to take up issues and discuss the implication of the exercise and plan action as a result.

In some homes the review highlighted problems in the staff group, but the general effect on staff morale was positive. It may be that opening up communication is necessary and beneficial in working through such problems—not talking about them will not make them go away. Some staff expressed initial anxiety about the work, but IQA generally provided a positive channel for discussion and development. In other cases, the review was experienced as a confirmation of good practice and increased staff confidence in looking at how improvements might be made.

Such effects were dependent to some extent, however, on how the review was conducted, for example, how well staff were prepared, consulted or involved in the work. It is early to make firm conclusions but there were indications from the comments of staff and managers that IQA will have an impact on the general attitudes of care workers towards the establishments, themselves as workers and towards residents as people.

Awareness of residents' needs and interests

One of the main results of the review was in beginning to question assumptions and attitudes and to shift the way staff thought about their work. The impact on staff attitudes can only be assumed or hoped to have a beneficial effect for residents but it is a view strongly backed by research evidence on institutional care (McCourt-Perring, 1993). In one case, a manager described the distress expressed by staff as they realised, for the first time, how residents felt about issues which had previously been closed or ignored—such as sexuality. Similarly, by being involved in the Quality Group, professionals came to see residents as people, like themselves. Responses from a number of homes suggested staff were more aware of residents' views in general and were, at times, surprised—even shocked—by the level and significance of their responses. It is encouraging that such learning was not generally seen as a threat but as an opportunity. The process and structure of the review gives staff the chance to participate and to own changes which may be needed.

Impact on Policy and Practice in Homes

Most managers responding to CESSA's questionnaire and to our interviews mentioned specific themes which had emerged for discussion and planning through the process. Not all had progressed as far as the formal report stage but most had specific plans and recommendations in mind. A number of managers found that things began to happen as a result of the activity itself with no need to wait for more formal planning. People expected the review to have an impact in several key areas.

First, the exercise exposed any lack of clarity regarding the aims and purposes of establishments. Many establishments involved did not have written aims and objectives, or needed to revise them since they were outdated. IQA provided an opportunity to involve a range of people in clarifying and stating these.

Second, the review heightened everyone's awareness of policy and resource issues. Noting points for change meant that people had to clarify who, and at what level in the agency, had power and responsibility to take action.

Third, the review report was a means of presenting information to the wider agency and outside interests. Several managers were keen to get messages across to senior officers. They considered that the report might well carry more weight than their own representations because residents' views were a major part of the review.

The changes which were reported to us included some small (but still important) changes in routines or environment—things which could be acted on in the short term and without major financial decisions. One home, for example, had introduced some choice in menus for the first time and had made some changes in room arrangements. Interestingly, one change had since been restored because the residents decided they preferred the original layout. More subtle changes were also apparent: after the review, visitors were greeted with a notice from the residents asking that they ring the bell and wait for a response before entering.

The review provided food for thought, and raised awareness of the issues to be tackled. Several managers were planning training activities as a follow up to the review. The experience of homes in the trial projects suggests that being involved—doing their own quality review—had helped establishments to change or to take a positive approach to change. One inspector, who had been involved in a quality group, commented that the home had made changes which had been suggested before but never fully acted upon.

The most frequently mentioned changes were material ones, which were perhaps the least challenging. The need for redecoration, new equipment, facilities or furniture was often raised. Minor alterations were often managed within home budgets, while those requiring larger funds were dependent on higher levels in the agency. Residents' comments were used by staff or managers to make a stronger case within their agency for added funds or facilities. The value of living and working in an environment which feels pleasant and cared for and of exercising choice should not be underestimated. These sort of changes were more commonly recognised and responded to than the issues relating to management, structure or policy although the symbolic value of physical improvements, however small and concrete, cannot be underestimated.

Our interviews also suggested that opening up communication can lead to change in the long term. A number of establishments had difficulties with barriers between different staff groups and between staff and residents, as well as difficulties in relation to the wider community. The dialogue involved in an IQA review was helpful in a number of ways. People began to learn more about each other and to communicate more openly. In some cases this also led to practice changes—such as the introduction of keywork or the creation of smaller living and working units within a large home. Similarly, a few developed plans for quite new ideas, such as creating special facilities for women within the home.

It was evident that some homes were struggling with the balance between individual and collective interests. One or two had hoped to use the review to feed into individual care planning but found it hard to do so and maintain confidentiality. Others felt unsure about how the interviews might link with formal complaints procedures without breaching confidentiality. One manager, for example, described feeling frustrated by a resident's request to have a bath on a different day, since she didn't know which resident it was. This reveals an underlying difficulty. The manager here, as elsewhere, had not considered the request as indicating a wider issue for the home: why not find out when all residents would prefer their bath? The majority of managers and staff seemed to lack a concept of how individual and collective matters might well be inter-related.

Several Quality Groups worked out how they would deal with complaints or individual requests. Interviewers were then able to discuss with residents how they could make a complaint or specific request. In one project, a serious complaint was made in an interview and was referred to an external manager. While this led to an immediate crisis of confidence in the Quality Group, the matter was openly discussed and led to the rethinking of certain guidelines and training for staff within the home.

Impact on Organisations

Impact on the wider organisation varied across projects but was generally minimal. Where the initial interest in IQA came from a senior officer, they retained an overview and were either involved in Quality Groups or kept in touch through updates and circulation of reports. A number of line managers had plans to try IQA with other establishments but few agencies had begun to consider how it might link in to operational areas like quality assurance or training. However, as review reports were only just beginning to circulate, it is early to assess how much impact the work might have on policies or procedures.

The experience in one development project highlights the limitations of IQA in affecting wider policy and practice if links with senior management are poor. The local authority took a keen interest in the request to participate and the home was involved in a pilot project and also undertook a full IQA review. The report was widely circulated and views from the home were positive. Although only limited changes were achieved, the staff were committed to a further review and were convinced of its value in moving the home forward. However, an inspection report during the period made no mention of the work. Line managers showed approval but little active interest and the pack was not taken up by other establishments in the authority. The department produced a policy document on quality assurance during this period, which mentioned quality action groups and interviewing residents—but made no reference to IQA. The overall impression was that awareness and interest was low, despite a conscious and current concern with quality. There was, it seemed, a difficulty to recognising the value and potential of grassroots experience for the agency as a whole.

In contrast, another SSD used IQA to develop a comprehensive quality assurance approach. The inspection unit was interested in how quality assurance might complement the inspection process and seconded one inspector to a Quality Group so that she could learn about the model. The unit had looked at the impact of residents' charters in all sectors and found them fairly ineffective: they were looking for ideas on how to involve lay people through advisory committees.

Many residential staff and managers felt isolated within their agencies and talked about lack of recognition or support. IQA had helped them to talk about these problems and to break down barriers between staff at different levels. At the same time, however, the experience shows how limited the influence of grassroots innovation can be if not supported by management and agency as a whole.

Impact on Outsiders and the Wider Community

Outsider members of Quality Groups had generally positive views. They saw the work as time consuming and demanding but rewarding. Several had changed their views about people who live in residential care and recognised the importance of enabling them to have a voice. One Quality Group chair—a manager of a different care home—found it opened up new perspectives about the needs and experience of people from different care groups. At first, he had been wary and rather dismissive, but IQA helped him to get to know the residents in a different way. Several home managers commented on the side benefit of developing new or closer links with people in the local community with an interest in the home.

Relatives were involved in the review through interviews and through participation in the Quality Group. In a number of homes, all relatives were sent questionnaires or interviewed by quality group members when visiting the home. More significant was the involvement of relatives in Quality Groups, which varied along care group lines and included parents (of young adults), spouses and daughters, sons or nieces of elders. It provided an opportunity for relatives to feel more positively involved with the establishment, as well as to express their views about the service offered to the person they cared for.

Discussion

One of the most signficant features of the IQA approach is that it concentrates on what people think and say. It is essentially a qualitative review using relatively simple tools. The appraisal of the home is based on personal and firsthand experience: external norms and standards are not introduced through detailed checklists or structured questionnaires.

The homes we visited indicated that this approach was welcomed and made sense to staff and residents alike. It was unintimidating, colloquial and allowed people to express *their* views and *their* ideas. Individual preoccupations came to the fore and enriched people's understanding and awareness of each other. Although residents tended to be sceptical about what could change, the interviews stimulated thought and opened up new possibilities of dialogue.

Arguably the most significant contribution of this research is in demonstrating that residents can participate: no care group was unable to respond given the opportunity and support to do so.

Using the IQA Review

Our evaluation indicates that the reviews carried out using the IQA pack have had positive results. These were certainly significant in individual homes where important, if small, changes took place. The fact that the majority of the trial homes intended to repeat the review shows the generally positive reception of IQA. The reasons for this were not only to do with the direct benefits to the home of, for example, appreciating the aspects which were working well and recognising those things which needed to change. People also felt positively about the system because it appealed to people's sense of fairness; it was workable, it involved people and incorporated a series of checks, balances and supports. Managers welcomed the opportunity to take the initiative without necessarily having to rely on wider agency support. Frontline staff, on the whole, responded well to the opportunity to participate and this was important in enabling them to feel some investment in the process and its outcomes.

This was the most successful of the CHI Programmes in involving residents directly. Not only did the work demonstrate how this could be done, it also showed there were benefits for residents from changes made in physical surroundings, in procedures and facilities and shifts in staff attitudes. There were also indirect benefits in that the review showed considerable potential for creating an atmosphere in which residents trust that they can speak out safely and be taken seriously.

Developing a climate in which people can express their views is potentially as important for staff as it is for residents. By advocating that each person is interviewed the system highlights the importance of the individual. This helps to offset any tendency to think about and respond to residents as a group and to deny that staff have valuable observations to make.

It seemed that the relative success of involving residents and, to a more limited extent, relatives and other outsiders, was due to the setting up of a specific structure—the Quality Group—which legitimates a series of activities which are distinct from the day-to-day management. Most of the work to date has been concerned with the operation of IQA within homes but project experience suggests that in-house reviews do have implications for the wider agency. It was clear, for example, that some of the action which homes wished to take would require support or resourcing from senior management but equally there may be important ways in which such a review could inform wider management policies and practices in relation to quality assurance.

IQA and Other Approaches to Quality Assurance

The work of IQA forms part of a wider development of and interest in approaches to quality assurance like quality circles or action groups (see for example Ward 1986), total quality management (see for example Oakland 1990) and the production of guidances and checklists for monitoring standards.

IQA is a development of a *quality action group* approach based on the idea of gathering together a small group of people who take responsibility for considering and reviewing quality issues. As we understand it, IQA is not unique in specifying the interests to be represented within the circle but the involvement of users is a recent development and not yet general practice. IQA may well be unique in making user views central to the review. It goes further than most in describing a system and tools which provide the opportunities and structures to ensure that individual views are obtained and that there is feedback to and from the different constituencies of interest.

Total quality management (TQM) has the aim of meeting customer requirements and, where possible, exceeding them. It is geared to ensuring that, throughout an organisation, workers and management understand the link between their work and the end point consumer of their services. Proponents see it as a philosophy within which all other mechanisms and tools can be integrated into a coherent organisation-wide approach. However, it is essentially a service-led model which relies most clearly on staff—administrators, managers and practitioners—taking the lead. It is not always specified how the customer—and other interest groups—are enabled to play a role in defining requirements or monitoring results and outcomes. We see it as a user-orientated approach but not one which requires, or specifically enables, direct user participation.

Checklist approaches, which we define in general terms as those which provide a systematic and comprehensive set of questions or aspects which can be considered and checked, have their limitations in ensuring that service users are centrally involved. We note, for example, that various guidelines developed by the Department of Health in implementation of community care make reference to the contribution which service users might make. However, prompting evaluators or inspectors to talk to residents or ask for their views does not tackle how this might be done. The work of Gibbs and Sinclair (1992) suggests that although checklists are an important aide memoire for inspectors, it is unhelpful to see these in terms of reaching a pass or fail score for a particular establishment. We note in our evaluation of the *'Home Truths'* booklet in Chapter 4 (Dawson et al, 1992) that checklists are welcomed but can lead to residents being the objects of the exercise rather than enabling their participation.

Certificated approaches are attractive to care home managers and proprietors because they lead to independent and externally recognised accreditation. BS 5750, the most widely known model, was used by a few establishments in the Initiative. It is a systematic approach which helps the individual establishment to define and set in place the procedures needed to carry out a quality review. What is subject to external validation, therefore, is whether or not a system of review has been set up (see Casson and George 1992). Accreditation is not based on an evaluation of standards and levels of service which have reference to established principles of good practice. BS 5750 does not embrace a particular set of values nor does it have any direct connection with residential care principles and practices. A critical gap in this approach is, therefore, that it does not necessarily challenge the objectives and standards which are determined by the service provider. Although many homes which have used BS 5750 have involved residents, the system does not require this.

We were made aware that external validation is of particular importance to care home managers and proprietors and many who valued IQA were looking for formal recognition. CESSA is currently pursuing the possibility of an IQA accreditation.

As we noted earlier, the significant way in which IQA differs from other approaches is the emphasis on qualitative and individual appraisal of service outputs. Impacts and outcomes are the experience of the service user and only they can comment on their level of satisfaction.

IQA, Quality of Service and Quality of Life

The significance of the IQA system is that it does not assume that notions of quality, of service standards or of quality of life are fixed or universal. The incorporation of different interests, and the views of different individuals and groups with a stake in how the home is run, means that the review and the actions which flow from it will always be the result of accommodation or negotiation between them. Notions of quality, good practice and priorities, will, to some extent, be defined and determined by successive reviews and the discussions which take place in between. A critical point is, therefore, whether the approach will prompt greater interaction and discussion among staff, between staff and residents, insiders and outsiders in the general day-to-day affairs of the establishment. Staff more than residents spoke to us about the changes in attitude and awareness which had taken place as a result of the review process and it seems likely that this kind of 'sea change' would be reinforced the more review and discussion involves residents and outsiders. What the system sets in place, therefore, is not a series of standards or definitions of quality but the people and constituencies of interest who are able to debate, define and implement these in relation to a particular home.

The relationships between in-house review, internal operational reviews and external systems of inspection and regulation were not systematically explored through the IQA trials. The system described by IQA is in some contrast to most approaches to self-evaluation which tend to be led by professional interests. Those who design and run the review are those who interpret the results. IQA, on the other hand, relies on the entry of a number of interests and is led by resident judgements. Inspectors and home managers considered that it would be important for IQA to remain as an in-house review, as a procedure distinct from, and independent of, external systems. However, inspectors who were involved in Quality Groups said they had learnt much from the experience, not only about the individual establishments but also about ways of promoting quality. There are some interesting points for development here. As inspection units establish their criteria and modes of work they show some divergence: some contribute to quality assurance by taking a developmental approach; others view the role as strictly to do with quality control and providing external judgements on standards of performance. In-house systems of review, like IQA, are clearly complementary to wider quality assurance measures but it is less clear in what way they might be linked to quality control.

Many care home managers saw considerable potential for using the report produced as a result of the IQA process in demonstrating the need for change or for action to senior management. The fact that residents had contributed to the review gave authority to the reports.

The effectiveness of all approaches to quality assurance depends on the extent to which they are legitimated and supported by the philosophy, policies and practices of the organisation. IQA, as a grassroots process of review, is able to secure bottom-up commitment but the work requires management support at higher levels in the agency if it is to lead to lasting change. There were some interesting, if small, indications that the power of frontline managers is increased when the voice of the resident is part of the review. The capacity of the grassroots to challenge strategic views and organisational goals will aways be limited but approaches like IQA play a part in extending the bases of participation.

Chapter 4

INFORMATION AND CHOICE

The importance of providing information for people seeking and using services was underlined by the Wagner review. The emphasis which it placed on the rights of the resident helped to highlight the essential role of information in underpinning choice for service users and ensuring that people know about their rights. There has been a growing understanding of the importance of information both to meet the internal requirements of service organisations and for service users. The intention of the new community care arrangements is to provide services on a needs-led and individual basis and this has led to recognition of the need for up-to-date and comprehensive information about the range and availability of care services in the community.

The provision of information is becoming a central concern of both purchasing and providing agencies but the kind of information—the content, format and availability—will differ according to the purposes of those who produce and disseminate it. This is a fundamental point. The distinction between the information dissemination needs of a service provider and the information requirements of potential service users is easy to lose sight of.

Providers need to promote knowledge of their services and to ensure that up-to-date, accurate and relevant information is available for purchasers, fund holders and service users. The format and distribution of information will differ according to the target groups. For example, there are considerable differences between advertising and promotional materials, comprehensive service information to support contract negotiations, information for management or financial audit and materials which inform people of their rights and eligibility for service.

Potential service users want information that is comprehensive, which addresses their questions, is accessible and which they can trust to be accurate. They also want information about how to obtain services, about alternatives and how to make comparisons and judgements between different possibilities.

Information, in whatever medium or format should, therefore, always be understood in relation to the intentions and purposes of those who produce and disseminate it, on the one hand, and those who receive and use it for their particular and perhaps different ends on the other.

The Policy Studies Institute was commissioned to look at provision of information as part of the Initiative. Originally this was to address the needs of people either in or considering a move into residential care. With the publication of the White Paper *Caring for People*, (HMSO, 1989b) and subsequent legislation, the objectives of the Programme were revised to address the much wider task of providing information for users of personal social services. The work, then, covered the macro-level of comprehensive information across a range of services and the micro-level of individual decision making between care options:

Information for users of personal social services

At the macro-level, the aim was to produce a comprehensive set of guidelines on how to tackle the practicalities of providing information for potential and current service users and their carers. The essential tasks were to understand the kind of information that people need, to identify means of collecting and making this available in ways that enable potential users to know which services are relevant to their needs and to make, where this is possible, informed choices between alternatives.

Information about residential care

At the micro-level the aim was, originally, to focus on the information needs of people considering or living in homes across the care groups.

The intention was to produce guidelines on the exchange of information needed to ensure that managers, residents and their carers are able to make well informed decisions. In the event, the booklet *Home Truths* (Dawson et al, 1992) addressed elderly people. It was developed through discussion with a number of care home managers and proprietors and written with them particularly in mind. We comment on this work later in the chapter.

We start by looking at the nature of the task of providing information about the wide range of care services for people in the community. We look at the scope of the Programme's work, the issues involved, the results of the pilot projects and the issues they raise about information provision.

Information for the Users of Personal Social Services

The emphasis of the work was on collating practical ideas and experience for setting up ways of providing information for users. There were two key features which shaped the work.

First, PSI was commissioned to design an approach which took the local authority Social Service Department (SSD) as the lead agency for establishing a system for gathering, collating and disseminating information. The reasons for this were twofold. SSDs have a responsibility for community care services (eg: in assessment, care and case management, purchasing and providing, inspecting) and therefore an intrinsic interest in gathering knowledge about the range and availability of services. The

Disabled Persons Act 1986, the Children Act 1989 and NHS & Community Care Act 1990 include a number of requirements that users of services receive good information, thus placing Social Service Departments in a key position in providing and ensuring this kind of information is available (Steele et al, 1993). SSDs were seen as agencies with the potential resources in time, money and strategic influence to set in place the policies, strategic planning, operating procedures, personnel (including inter-agency links and securing the collaboration of other agencies) and technology required.

The second feature was that the researchers tackled the task on an issue-by-issue basis. The practical projects which were set up explored particular aspects of information provision but these were not located within an overall frame of the essential elements of a system and the operational links between them. A prototype system was not developed in the way that, for example, the CESSA team prepared a trial IQA pack. The research was conducted in a series of independent, theme based projects linked by the overall task.

The Value Base
The values which underpinned the work were clearly stated and linked to the notion that access to appropriate information is essential in exercising choice:

> 'If (information) is to lead to optimum and appropriate decisions it must be:
> - accurate and up-to-date
> - objective and independent
> - comprehensive
> - accessible and comprehensible.'   (PSI, 1989)

These values implicitly endorse the rights and interests of the service user: the PSI approach thus embraced a user orientation that was entirely consistent with the Wagner review and the other Programmes. Even though the work was more concerned with strategic level planning than that of direct service within an individual care home, the basic principles of understanding and meeting the interests of the consumer were the same.

The Context for Developing Information Provision
In developing guidelines on providing information for users of personal and social care services, across the voluntary, private and statutory sectors, the PSI team was faced with a considerable task. There were several aspects to this.

The changing foundations of community care services
The fundamental changes in community care services that were taking place during the life of the CHI have already been outlined. In relation to

the work of the PSI, however, it is important to note that any move to provide information for users of the personal social services was taking place in a fast changing environment. In some respects, this affected the work of PSI more than the other Programmes. Whereas other researchers were working with individual care establishments, the work of information provision spanned potentially, not only the SSD as an organisation but also the main lines of connection between it and other agencies.

We noted earlier that the new legislation makes requirements about the provision of information and places the rights and needs of users firmly on the agenda. All providers have the same responsibility to ensure that they disseminate information for users and potential users of their services.

Information cultures

The collation and use of information within service organisations has been largely confined to financial data and service statistics—often shaped by the requirements of central government departments. Wider information provision and use in the field of care services have not, until recently, been recognised as essential elements in the internal functioning of service organisations although the setting up of internal systems has been expanding rapidly. In this context, providing information specifically to meet the requirements of service users embraces a relatively new set of ideas and involves a shift in emphasis and focus on the part of provider agencies.

Our interviews with SSD personnel at all levels and independent sector agencies participating in CHI confirmed that, whereas *information for the internal purposes* of the organisation was becoming an established part of setting up, managing and monitoring services, there was little spontaneous discussion or recognition of the *information needs of service users*. The agencies participating in the PSI projects were aware of and planning for user needs but even here the primary concern—the motivation for engaging time and personnel—was to disseminate accurate information *about the services* provided by that agency in the new era of community care. In five of the SSDs running pilot projects with PSI there were strong indications that, even where the objectives clearly stated a user focus, their interests were debated almost exclusively in terms of what SSD staff considered that users needed to know about SSD services and procedures, and the new legislation.

These observations suggest that it is difficult for all agency personnel, but particularly staff in SSDs, to establish a clear user orientation. The difference between internal information systems and those which provide information for the use and benefit of service users has to be understood if users are to obtain information that is useful and relevant to them.

Information as a practice and management resource: SSDs

We asked people at different levels in SSDs across the Programmes about the ways in which information was handled and used in their department.

The picture is necessarily partial but the comments suggested the same broad situation. Typically, information or knowledge is power: it is acquired in specific ways from particular people and shared with others for particular purposes. We were told that information tends to be gathered and used in particular ways by the different functional areas within a SSD (eg. finance, training and recruitment, operational management, information about service recipients): people do not think about the information needs of the organisation as a whole. The tendency is to treat information as currency with potential trading value rather than an open resource which can be made available and used by all.

It is usually assumed that information flows down from the top. As one SSD respondent put it 'information comes from the top: it rarely gets below middle management because people hang on to it. Information is power—it divides those in the know from others.'

Equally people referred to a cut-off point in relation to information moving up a department. There is a level beyond which information from the operational units and frontline workers is not interesting or legitimate unless specifically requested by higher management.

It has not been usual for SSDs to share information with externals. Some of the difficulties of joint health and social service collaboration have arisen from failures to communicate effectively about policies, priorities, resources and working practices. Lateral information flow, especially that which crosses organisational boundaries, tends to follow traditional and well established routes at senior levels: these have not, typically, involved private or voluntary sector agencies, nor has inter-agency discussion been encouraged at grassroots. We noted how isolated individual care establishments can be: discussions with peers in other homes did not appear to be the norm in SSDs.

A defensive attitude in SSDs
Although attitudes to information usage are changing our observations suggest that there is an underlying defensiveness in many SSDs about providing information for the general public. There were several facets to this:

- in many cases policies and priorities were described as poorly defined and understood within the department. In these situations it is almost impossible for staff to describe or explain eligibility for service, access or assessment procedures accurately;

- linked with this was a general anxiety about the possible consequences—for the individual or the department—of misrepresentation;

- there was a fear that providing more information would increase demand for services;

• people also spoke of, or implied, a personal confusion of loyalty about how to deal with poor or inadequate levels of service: should they protect their SSD from outside criticism? or speak out for better services for the user?

How SSDs are perceived by other organisations

Our contacts across a large number of voluntary, private, user and carer organisations indicated a widespread scepticism about the capacity of SSDs to provide and purchase a comprehensive or integrated range of services. Equally SSDs have played a relatively minor role in service provision for some groups—in the fields of mental health, drug and alcohol and physical disability, for example. Not surprisingly representatives of these care groups questioned the role of the SSD in future developments. They pointed out that new relationships would have to be forged before an effective exchange of information could be established between the agencies involved.

Many specialist voluntary agencies have a tradition of collating and disseminating information on rights and services for their particular client or user group and could see the SSD as a potential customer for such knowledge.

The needs of different care groups

The information needs of users of personal social and care services span a very wide range of provision relevant to the different care groupings.

All groups with which we have had contact confirmed the essential role that information can play in ensuring people have access to the services they require or, at least, have knowledge of the gaps and what is not available (Perring, 1991).

Our observations, from this and other Programmes, suggest that although there are no fundamental technical or practical differences to be taken into account for different care groups, there are important communication, access and credibility issues to be understood.

Communication issues include those relating to language, style, presentation and medium: the PSI Programme collated some general material on these aspects (Lewis 1990) but some groups do have specific needs:

Discovering the best means of reaching and communicating with, for example, people with learning disabilities, children, black and ethnic minority groups or people with visual/hearing impairment, implies the need for specialised approaches that are informed by the users concerned.

Access issues include availability, location and timing. Questions about centralised versus local means of disseminating information may have different answers according to care group. How far does information need to be specifically timed and targeted in order to reach certain people? Such questions can only be answered by having a good understanding of the experience, patterns of need, and the typical career paths of people requiring help.

Credibility issues relate to the extent that people see the SSD or any agency or system as an acceptable, reliable and credible source of help, service or information. There is a lot of evidence to suggest that very few people would consider SSDs an appropriate source of information. For example, people with particular difficulties whose needs have not been a central part of SSD service provision—like those with mental health, drug and alcohol problems—are unlikely to seek help from a SSD-led information service. Equally families and parents with child care needs are likely to view SSDs with caution.

Equally, there is a great deal of evidence to show that black people and those from ethnic minority groups have little confidence in white-run institutions and organisations and those with few, if any, staff from their own racial and cultural background. They are less aware of SSD services and have fewer connections with the main networks of information and advice (Swarup, 1992).

The Challenge

The policy and organisational contexts within which the work was developed were, therefore, complex and challenging. A comprehensive system of information provision that reaches and is relevant for service users would have to tackle the following series of points:

- ensuring that the format, content and dissemination of information is determined by users' views and needs;

- the provision of comprehensive information of this sort requires collaboration between a wide range of agencies, service providers and other sources of relevant information. The system would have to incorporate cross-agency and cross-sector communication and challenge traditional attitudes to sharing and opening up access to information;

- providing information should be seen as an integral part of providing a service and, therefore, the responsibility of all;

- those providing information would need guidance in understanding that the kind of information which is useful and relevant for the general public and specific users may differ, in important respects, from the information that they might wish to provide for their own purposes;

- the SSD—or any lead agency or information network—requires the resources—finances, policy backing, staffing—to collate and disseminate information, to secure the collaboration of a wide constituency of users and providers and to set in place the necessary infrastructure and technology.

The Programme's Work

Early work by the team looked at the *underlying issues* (Steele 1990) and finding out about the *information needs of services users* and how they seek information (Roberts et al 1990).

A survey of written information provided by local authorities and residential care agencies was carried out, analysed and published as *guidance on presentation and information design* (Lewis 1990).

A *Consultative Group* was convened to provide a forum for discussion, information and practice exchange. This consisted of representatives from twelve SSDs selected because they had made progress in developing systems for providing user information. The SSDs included a range of shire and metropolitan authorities, political characteristics and geographical location.

The Group included people with experience of a system based on a comprehensive audit of services available by client group across the authority; a system based on setting up information access points linked to GP surgeries; partial moves towards a collaborative system with user groups; a federation/agency network approach. The Group also included an action researcher concerned with the development of information networks for people with physical disability.

Pilot projects were set up in collaboration with six of the SSDs on the Consultative Group. The aims and focus of these were decided in two ways. The Consultative Group identified a series of aspects of information provision which the researchers then explored in practice. Most of these coincided with the interests of particular SSDs who were then able to pursue these with help from the PSI in a series of pilot projects.

Each project was supported by a member of the PSI team whose role varied somewhat depending on the type of project and the objectives of the pilot authority. In most cases they acted as catalysts for action as well as working directly with local staff in conducting surveys and interviews, writing materials, contributing to meetings. They also provided information, ideas, feedback and access to other groups but did not, on the whole, provide leadership for the projects: this was taken by local staff usually with their own working or advisory group. The focus, resourcing and pace of the projects was, therefore, largely in local hands.

The range of aspects covered by the projects was extensive but not necessarily comprehensive since they were not related to an overall framework identifying of the key elements for providing information for users. The pilot SSDs received a copy of a preliminary paper prepared by the PSI team which addressed a series of practical, action-orientated questions. This provided a structure for planning the projects but did not indicate how they might link together. Each project group worked independently drawing on the experience of the PSI and other SSDs.

A two-day seminar for the Consultative Group and the researchers was held to discuss the draft guidelines that were produced following the projects.

In all, thirteen projects were set up in six LA/SSDs although not all were completed. The work included services for elders, children, people with learning disabilities and those with physical disabilities. People with mental health, drug or alcohol problems were not represented.

The pilot authorities agreed to work with the PSI consultants over a six month period. The time frame was geared to the production of draft guidelines in early 1992 but most planned to continue after contact with PSI had ended.

The range of pilot work

The following list of projects shows something of the range of issues which were identified as relevant and important:

- information provision to black and ethnic minority communities: an interview-based investigation into the views and needs of these groups, their patterns of information seeking, and relationships with the SSD;

- information provision to professionals and other agencies: for example, a survey-based assessment of the use made of a Resource Directory, plus some interviews with GPs;

- information and training for reception and frontline staff;

- consultation with users and carers: how to improve information exchange between users, carers, service providers and the SSD based on surveys, interviews and meetings with representatives from selected groups;

- dissemination in rural areas: an investigation based on interviews in four rather different rural communities;

- information needs and priorities of the SSD: an internal investigation based on interviews with strategic and operational staff on the information implications of existing policies and new legislation;

- providing information about new care management systems for elderly people;

- developing a departmental strategy for providing information to users of social services in the county;

- information and children's services: how comprehensive information on the Children Act might be made available and acceptable/relevant for children, parents and others;

- information for people with learning disabilities: a working group involved user and carer groups to consider what information existed, was needed and to explore different means of communicating.

The projects thus covered a number of different concerns ranging across geographical, care group, communication, strategic planning and resource considerations. They also varied between work intended to help the SSD put out information about its own services and arrangements, work focused on finding out about the needs of users, and work at a more systematic level looking at patterns of information dissemination.

None of the projects set out to integrate these different aspects or to implement a full system but each was expected to contribute to the overall thinking of the SSD concerned and to act as a catalyst for further development.

We can note, therefore, that although the PSI acquired practical information the experience was individual, context specific and difficult to translate into general notions and practical approaches. It was also the case that the projects involved work only with and within SSDs: no direct work with other agencies and organisations was undertaken.

Learning from the Projects

From the SSDs' point of view, the projects were seen as partial approaches which would help to establish the importance of information provision for service users as well as achieving specific outcomes. Individual authorities learnt from the experience and all continued to develop work in the area of information provision after the end of PSI involvement. What follows is a brief account of the main issues which emerged from the pilot work.

Key People

Most of the work was led by people either in middle management or in staff roles. The projects provided them with valuable experience in thinking about user information alongside the tasks of community care implementation. The links between service provision and user needs were thus highlighted and so formed the basis—however small—of a more integrated understanding of the need for and purposes of information.

The commitment of the people leading the projects and their interest in information provision made the most difference to the progress and results of the work: although many did not have the authority to set in place new procedures, their knowledge and enthusiasm certainly helped to ensure that issues concerning information were kept on the agenda. As information has become a more political issue in meeting charter and rights requirements, these people were recognised as having experience and knowledge which could be more actively utilised. The involvement of the PSI consultants, as with other CHI projects, added authority to the projects which helped to establish the importance of the work internally.

The Validity of Providing Information for Users

The pilot projects took place in local authorities where the responsibility of the SSD in providing information for users had been accepted in principle. However, the extent to which the work was accepted as having some priority varied considerably. On the whole the projects were operating at the margins of other aspects of SSDs' work. For example, some projects were financed because of the necessity of informing the public about complaints procedures. In one, materials were prepared to inform people about the new assessment and care management arrangements—a central operational change—but the work was paid for, not from an operational budget, but from a small amount of money made available by the information officer involved in the pilot project.

The general message was that information work was valid but of low value when competing with operational issues. In most cases it was narrowly defined as information that the SSD had a responsibility to provide about its own services and procedures. By the end of our evaluative work there were indications that authorities were prepared to give more priority to information provision but with emphasis on their own services, rather than meeting user requirements.

A User Orientation

Apart from two projects there was a marked tendency to see and talk of the service user as a recipient of information. Although several project groups spoke of users' needs there was no sustained commitment to inviting their views or including user organisations in planning meetings. The general tenor of the work fell into the category of informing people about the work and services of the SSD. Although it was recognised that people require knowledge of alternatives in order to make choices, the actual plans and work did not maintain this orientation. However, the issue of taking the users' point of view and the benefits of consultation with user groups were strong themes in the two-day workshop of the Consultative Group.

Two projects did explore information needs from the users' point of view. In one, a detailed survey was carried out to establish the needs of rural and dispersed populations and how the SSD might meet these. Customer services staff carried out a questionnaire survey, interviewed local people and agencies in a number of areas and canvassed the views of SSD personnel in order to obtain a picture of information needs, networks and priorities. The approach was questioning and open to new ideas.

Another project involved people with learning disabilities. User groups and individuals were invited to explore the kind of information that people with learning disabilities and their families needed and different ways of making this available. The project group tried theatre, video and role play techniques, all involving users themselves. The work was important, not only because it achieved some direct results in terms of information shared and valuable relationships set up, it also revealed to those involved the slow and sensitive nature of working in collaboration with user groups.

Internal Policy

Several projects where the aim was to produce information for the public about SSDs' own services found their work hampered by the lack of internal clarity about policies, priorities and eligibility for services. One project group took a considerable amount of time to ensure that the wording on a pamphlet was accurate without implying that all who were eligible could, as a right, obtain a particular service. The level of anxiety about misrepresentation at a time of reduced levels of service showed clearly how the provision of information to the public can run into political issues. SSD personnel were—or felt—unable to inform the public about actual service levels. This group, and others, were able to voice their concerns and draw attention to the need for careful thought about people's right to information.

Developing an Information Strategy

Although the projects pursued particular aspects of information provision, all agreed it was essential that the SSDs established a policy on information. In some cases an information strategy had been adopted but these usually concerned internal information handling and use. The issues covered related to the information needs of the organisation within which, if they featured at all, user requirements were a marginal aspect of operational or service management. Internal strategies tended to be dominated by issues about technological systems and their compatibilities rather than specifying the nature and purposes of collecting, disseminating, accessing and using information. It was not surprising, therefore, that progress in the pilot projects towards the formulation of an overall SSD strategy for users was generally slow.

During our follow-up work, however, there was evidence that the implementation of care management systems was highlighting the need for better information across the range of services. In one case, a key member of the project group who had been pushing for a user information strategy for over two years found that cautious acceptance had changed into high profile commitment at senior level.

Time Scales

Most of the projects took longer than anticipated. The duration was obviously related to the amount of time that staff could give to the work but the commitment of project workers and their seniority also made a difference.

One of the most time-consuming activities for staff within the SSD was agreeing the content, style and format of information leaflets and other materials for public distribution.

The few projects which involved other agencies found the time taken to convene meetings and agree plans extended the time scale. A significant, but not surprising, finding from the project which most successfully involved service users, was the considerable amount of time needed for real consultation, sharing ideas and reflecting on the results with a range of other people.

Costs and Resources

Given the partial nature of the projects it was not possible to assess the kind of costs involved in setting up and running a comprehensive system. The issue was discussed by Consultative Group members and their experience suggested a number of aspects of cost and resource that would have to be borne in mind.

There was agreement that the major cost would be that of staffing. Whatever system was adopted it would need dedicated staff and this would mean, depending on the size of the authority, at least the appointment of a full-time officer with specific responsibility for user information. It was felt that, since information should be an intrinsic part of service provision, the cost of suitable materials and keeping front line staff up to date within the organisation should be costed into operational budgets. The cost of technology would depend very much on the extent to which the system might be based in computerised data handling. Opinions were somewhat divided about the extent to which information technology could deliver the kind of interactive system necessary to cope with the amount of contact and networking between an information unit located within the social service department and sources of information like provider agencies, user groups, information and advice centres.

Some departments had considered the issue on the basis of a percentage of total revenue and some believed that start-up costs would be the most significant feature. After that, costs could be more or less absorbed within general financing of services.

Learning from the Work as a Whole

From the projects the PSI team produced a set of draft guidelines for discussion with the Consultative Group in a two-day workshop. A number of issues emerged from this and some of these we discuss now.

Ideas About the Kind of System Required

The kind of system required to collect information about an extensive range of services, across sectors of provision and care groups and to make this available and accessible to a highly diverse population of potential users is complex.

We found a high level of agreement that such a system:

- requires strategic planning and commitment;

- should be understood as a process involving feedback and interaction between the different elements;

- should include information for other professionals and advisers as well as service users and their families;

- should provide alternative means of dissemination;

- should involve collaboration between service providers and users.

Content and Philosophy of an Information Strategy for Users

The ideas discussed during the workshop endorsed an analysis of information strategies which had been carried out earlier by the PSI team. There was a broad consensus that:

- a cultural shift in organisations was needed (not only SSDs) in which information is seen as an essential part of service provision;

- everyone involved in providing a service has a responsibility for providing information;

- information provision should be user-led: i.e. by those who need and use information not by the characteristics of the equipment or technology;

- that there are important training implications for managing information;

- staff need to be well informed in order to inform users.

Consumer or User Orientation

Several important aspects which emerged from our interviews with user organisations and which were confirmed in the PSI survey of users (Roberts et al, 1990) suggest that:

- most people seek information from other people;

- the value of the information obtained is strongly linked with how the information giver is viewed: their credibility and reliability becomes a measure of the value and accuracy of the information they impart;

- people often need advice on *how* to obtain information;

- they often require help to use information to make decisions;

- people want to know about the quality of a service: they seek value judgements and comparisons;

- people want information about their rights

Providing information *for service users* was seen, therefore, as an undertaking requiring a particular approach to the way information is collected.

Information Cultures

There was a recognition that ideas about handling and using information were undergoing a cultural shift and one which was necessary if agencies were to take on the task of ensuring that their users were well informed. The essence of the shift was from thinking about the capacities of machines to appreciating the kind of information people need for particular purposes. Table 4.1 summarises the shift in values which are consistent with this new thinking: those involved in the Consultative Group and people we interviewed across CHI broadly endorsed these ideas.

TABLE 4.1—Cultural Shifts Required to Support Information Provision for Service Users

From:	To:
An emphasis on technology and the way information is *stored and handled*	Designing systems that take account of the way information is *used* by people
The use of mathematical computing and handling hard facts	Using computer graphics, visual display, and concrete images that are are accessible to people with no computing skills or knowledge
Designing technical systems: linkages and characteristics of the equipment	Understanding people and patterns of living; their networks and interactions and information needs
Concern to ensure efficient *output* of materials	Concern with *uptake*: using and adapting to informal patterns and networks to ensure information reaches people
Avoiding duplication	Using a variety of information and methods to convey the message and ensure uptake
Focus on service management requirements	Focus on service use and service user requirements

---

The Guidelines Produced

The guidelines, *Informing People About Social Services* (Steele et al, 1993) are published in four parts, each addressing a different audience and tackling different tasks. They are styled as a package of guidance for SSDs on developing information services for users and the public.

'Meeting the Need for Information'

This part addresses directors of SSDs and elected members. It sets out the reasons why an information strategy is needed and why the SSD has a responsibility to meet legislative requirements and general needs in this area. The guide emphasises that the public and potential service users have a right to good information in terms of entitlement and knowledge of alternatives. It refers to a general trend towards greater consumer participation and control through initiatives like the Patient's Charter.

The issue of limited resources and resulting cautions about providing service information is acknowledged but the guide comments:

> 'The failure to inform people about services is hard to justify as it results in a system where services are rationed through ignorance when they should be allocated according to need.'

> (Steele et al, 1993)

The guide takes a clear line, therefore, that the provision of information is for the benefit of potential and actual service users.

'The User Information Policy'

Part Two provides guidelines for policy makers and senior management on the formulation of a comprehensive approach to setting up a system of information provision. The elements of a policy are itemed and some of the key features of the system are identified. For example, the guide advocates that management and user information services should be integrated and that the system should serve those who need and use information rather than be determined by the technology.

The guide identifies the different groups of people who will need information—the general public, potential and actual service users, carers and relatives and those who are 'unwilling users' like children in care, other professionals and other service providers and points out that they should be consulted about their information requirements.

A section on working with other organisations refers to the need for SSDs to work jointly with, and obtain information about, other services and information providers. The guide does not emphasise, however, the essential aspect of collating comprehensive information to cover the needs of the wide range of care groups and their interests. The advice to set up a working group to steer the development of a policy mentions, but does not strongly advocate, the involvement of agencies and people from outside the SSDs.

'Developing Information Services For Users'

Part Three is a practical guide for those involved in setting up and running a system. The guide advocates that a central information unit and clearing house is established

> 'to co-ordinate and facilitate information work throughout the department and to liaise with external information providers and other agencies' (Steele et al, 1993)

and that its remit should be authority wide.

The guide refers to the need for appropriate training for information work—to cover knowledge of sources, handling and interpreting information, methods of dissemination and presentation—and in aspects of communication. The roles of receptionists and frontline staff are identified as of particular importance in responding to people's need for information.

The resource implications are discussed in relation to the overall view that everyone in the organisation has a part to play in providing good information and that this should became an integral part of service provision. The main resource implications are staffing and equipping an information unit and the costs of printing and dissemination.

The guidelines also tackle some of the practical issues of auditing and verifying existing information, sorting out the kind of data needed, how and from where it can be collected, methods of updating and handling qualitative information. A section here refers to the need to obtain the co-operation of and to work with users, voluntary and private sector agencies, other departments of the local authority, the health authority and national sources of information.

A final section discusses practical aspects of getting the message across: for example, thinking about the needs of different groups, how to reach rural communities and people with special needs, using different means of providing information, designing materials, mapping possible outlets and contacts, using the media.

'The Summary of Legislation and Guidance'

Part Four is a comprehensive listing of recent legislation and central guidances as these refer to, or have application for, information provision.

Discussion

In summary we comment on the extent to which the published guidelines address the issues that have been raised and describe effective ways of meeting the needs of service users.

The guidelines provide a systematic and clear set of procedures for SSDs to set in place the policies, resources and practice arrangements for providing information. They guide readers through various levels of decision making and identify, in a number of ways, how providing information for service users differs from meeting internal requirements.

They reflect a strong orientation to understanding and meeting the needs of people who use services and prompt everyone, from councillors to senior managers and frontline workers, to consider their role in ensuring that information is available and relevant.

As such, the guides represent an important point in the history of service provision in recognising the rights and needs of the public for good information and the role that a statutory agency can play. The guidelines are authoritative to the extent that they address the particular circumstances of SSDs.

But there are also important respects in which the guidelines fall short of a comprehensive approach that fully addresses user interests.

The advice is confined, almost entirely, to the internal arrangements of the SSD. The guidelines include reference to the importance of working with other agencies and incorporating the knowledge and views of service users. But they do not envisage the kind of practical arrangements that such collaboration might require. They say nothing, for example, about the mechanisms and relationships that might be needed and they do not identify the kind of existing networks that could be used.

Setting up collaborative structures and opportunities is treated as unproblematic throughout. There is no discussion about the potential difficulties to be anticipated and planned for, although a number of issues did emerge from the projects and Consultative Group discussions. One of these, for example, concerned the way that SSD personnel tend to dominate meetings intended to ensure the participation of a range of agencies.

The role of other organisations is not considered in that the guidelines do not identify and suggest an active agenda for the other agencies and institutions that might be important contributors in designing and running a system that is comprehensive. The intention of the NHS and Community Care Act 1990 is to make the integration of services possible and this means closer understanding and collaboration between health and social care services, between statutory and independent providers.

An important issue, since the ideas are framed with SSDs in mind, is the tendency throughout for the advice to conflate information *about SSD services* and information *for users*. Although the orientation towards the requirements of users is clearly stated, the practical measures to ensure that this is recognised and maintained are weak. Again, there is no discussion or illustration that prompts people to recognise the difference between traditional ways of thinking about information and the new, open culture required to meet user needs.

The guides do not discuss aspects of information provision which help to ensure that what people receive is more than facts and data. People often require advice about how to use information, advocacy in recognising their rights and pressing for them, education about how systems and services work. These are tasks which SSD professionals have been reluctant to take on and for which they may themselves need to acquire specialist knowledge.

Linked with this is a final point. People want to make choices, where these exist, based on judgements and comparisons. Advice and guidance as to the quality and value of a service, judgements about reliability and effectiveness are the kind of help people seek. Clearly these are activities that could conflict with the general expectations (and requirements) that SSDs are even-handed. The role of advice and specialist voluntary agencies has always been stronger in this area and their participation in information provision would seem essential.

These gaps appear to us to stem from the design features which we referred to earlier: in taking the SSD as the lead agency there was no exploration of possible alternative strategies; individual projects were undertaken which had little reference to each other; there was no overall approach or model used to help identify and explore the key tasks and elements involved in providing information for services users. There was, then, no shared understanding of the key interest groups, agencies and systems within which care services are provided and the pros and cons of taking SSDs as the lead agency.

Alternative Approaches and the Way Forward

An unintended difficulty is that the guides might be taken to signal that the SSD has a sole responsibility for tackling information provision or that they are the only agency with the resources to do so. This is clearly not the case: many care group and user organisations have taken the lead for years in providing specialist information. National and local specialist sources will continue to be essential for different care group and user interests. Facilities for people with drug or alcohol related problems, for example, cover a wide, if not national, catchment area. Services for people with mental health problems cover different professions and agencies across health and social services.

One of the central problems, as we see it, relates to the knowledge of local, formal and informal facilities which support people living in the community. The issue is complex: it is about the realities of life for, and aspirations of, the individual. The rhetoric of care management is that services will be co-ordinated to meet the particular needs of the individual. Leaving aside the issue of the costs involved, there is a prior and fundamental question about how knowledge of the facilities and opportunities that exist can be accessed. Much of the thinking about community care services has, inevitably, centred on elders. But if we think about the needs of the younger adult with physical disabilities, the range of potential services or facilities about which information is required increases: for example, accommodation, social, leisure, educational and work opportunities, transport facilities. The relevant agencies to meet these needs might span private, voluntary, commercial and public sectors: who holds the knowledge about what can be provided and, equally important, which agency might be encouraged to meet user demands?

Such questions point to the need for detailed, local knowledge. Is this part of the remit of SSD care managers? It was an aspect that the PSI project touched on in relation to rural communities but not in relation to specific care groups. The PSI is currently working with twelve federations—cross-sector alliances of agencies concerned with the needs of people with physical and mental health disabilities—as part of the National Disability Information Project. These federations are taking on the work of collecting and disseminating information for their area. The areas covered are quite large—for example a metropolitan borough, a shire county, a large rural area—but they include groups and agencies operating in small local areas. One of the aspects of information provision on which the work will provide information is how local and detailed information needs to be to meet individual needs and how far it has to incorporate national provision.

Federations are, we understand, springing up and surviving in all parts of the country and it will be important to evaluate how successful these innovations can be in meeting user information requirements.

Another model of information provision is that of the voluntary agency set up to provide a case management service for a particular group of people. The care management service CHOICE, run by and for people with physical disabilities in the London Borough of Barnet is an example. Such an agency would complement a SSD-led strategy. Here the task of defining needs and the best way of meeting these is tackled by the individual concerned and a worker. The organisation collects information about facilities, services, knowledge about policies and priorities, eligibility and access, about standards and service providers' track records. An issue which this kind of agency can address, in some measure, is that of providing the kind of qualitative information people are looking for in deciding between alternatives.

We noted the different traditions of service and wide variation in the extent to which potential service users are active, organised, even campaigning in ensuring that their needs are known about and addressed. Service providers and information networks could find a valuable source of information, guidance and advice in user-run and user-led organisations.

Information about Residential Care for Elderly People

The Department of Health also commissioned the Policy Studies Institute to produce guidelines on the provision of information for people entering or living in residential establishments. This was a small-scale undertaking as an adjunct to the work on providing information for users of social services. It was intended to identify, and provide practical guidelines on, the role of information provision and exchange in helping to ensure that users, potential users and their carers can make effective decisions about residential care services.

The guidelines were to have addressed the needs of all the care groups included in the CHI work but, with limited time available, the researchers focused on information for elderly people. These are published as a booklet, *Home Truths* (Dawson et al, 1992).

Many of the fundamental issues relating to the provision of information are the same at micro- and macro-levels but in focusing on the needs of the individual rather than the aggregated requirements of users, the work looked at particular issues about timing and the processes of exchange.

Development of the Guidelines

The researchers began by asking a number of care home managers and proprietors from a range of fifteen establishments for elders about their current practice and about information needs. They also drew on earlier Programme work on information needs (Steele, 1990; Roberts et al, 1990).

From these enquiries the team produced draft guidelines which were discussed further with care home managers and amended in the light of their feedback and suggestions. Some discussions were also held with other CHI researchers about the needs of elders and the PSI team had access to many of the working papers and reports of the Programmes.

What the guidelines cover

The guidelines are structured around different points in the process of selecting and entering a care establishment. Sections cover:

- the initial enquiry from a potential resident or their carer: this covered the kind of information required by people making decisions about care and service alternatives and by managers making assessments about someone's suitability for their home;

- the process of admission covering visits to the resident's own home, visits to the establishment by the resident and trial stays: this covered the kind of information needed by both resident and care staff;

- the continuing information needs of the resident during the first month in a residential home: the documents: brochures, residents' handbooks and contracts—the kind of information people need in continuing care.

An Appendix provides checklists and information materials which can be photocopied.

Responses to *Home Truths*

In order to obtain views on the usefulness of the guidelines and comments on the practice it describes, we conducted a questionnaire survey of people who had purchased *Home Truths*, visited and interviewed managers, staff and residents in six homes for elders and a number of senior managers, trainers and inspectors. In addition we asked representatives of a number of organisations for elderly people, their relatives and carers for their views and comments on the guidelines (Appendix 1.5).

The comments we obtained fell into three main categories.

General approach
The guidelines were generally welcomed and seen as an important contribution to improving service quality. The overall approach was considered helpful but limited. The emphasis on checklists and itemising information to be collected or provided detracted from a consideration of the principles involved and the broad purposes of the exchange. It was felt, for example, that the interests of the home, the management and staff were dominant and that the materials tended not to prompt careful attention to the situation of the prospective resident.

There was a tendency to confuse and conflate three different tasks:

• providing information for prospective residents, their relatives and carers about the home and about alternative services, as an aid to decision making;

• obtaining information from the potential resident as a way of ensuring that they are suitable and meet the home's eligibility criteria;

• exchanging detailed information at the point of admission—ie after a decision has been taken, at least for a trial stay—to build a good understanding between home and resident about their needs and what the home has to offer.

Part of the intention of the guidelines is to help people to make informed choices and this implies knowledge of alternatives. It is doubtful that care home managers and proprietors could ever be in a position to provide detailed, accurate and unbiassed information about other homes or services but the guidelines do provide a leaflet that managers can send to enquirers about how to approach the business of selecting a care home.

Content
The content was seen as fair and detailed and, as a check on the kind of information required at each stage, a helpful tool in hand. However, most of the people we interviewed considered that the content was limited in important ways.

First there was a strong bias towards the information to be collected from the individual elderly person. The content generally gave most emphasis to the details that were required by the home. In doing so the guidelines were seen as having a somewhat mechanistic approach to a series of highly important meetings between people. Respondents, especially those representing organisations for elderly people, carers and relatives, wanted more attention to be given to the way people were seen and the quality of the relationship established during the process.

Second, respondents thought the guidelines concentrated on medical history and physical incapacity and had a general problem orientation: the abilities, aspirations, social relationships, emotional needs and interests of the elderly person were either not covered or addressed in a negative way. It is, however, unfair to see this as a criticism of these guidelines. They are by no means unusual in taking this approach: they reflect the kind of practice in many establishments which is strongly shaped by medical and nursing traditions of care. The overall effect is that elderly people do not appear to be seen as whole individuals but as a package of problems and details to be recorded and dealt with.

Third, respondents pointed out that the guidelines do not prompt people to think about the context within which the exchange of information was taking place. The process is taken as unproblematic although, in reality, people are usually considering a move into a home in a state of crisis and considerable emotional upheaval. As increasingly people enter a residential establishment from hospital the process of entry is very different from that assumed by *Home Truths*. The implementation of care management means, in any case, that assessment for care needs and much of the preliminary discussion will have taken place, in many cases, before a home manager is involved.

Format and style
The format of the booklet and the use of checklists prompted a number of comments. Many people liked the detailed points and lists and considered these useful ways of ensuring that important issues are not overlooked. But more people were concerned that this kind of approach can give a false sense of security—of having covered the ground effectively because all the items have been considered. It can act against careful discussion of individual and idiosyncratic needs and wishes. Many of the representatives from organisations for elderly people and their carers were irritated by the detail—which some found patronising.

It was a measure of the success of the guide that several people referred to particular points about presentation and style. The print size was too small some felt and many found the lay-out too wordy and dense. Many looked for illustrative materials and scenes from practice as a way of highlighting issues and helping people to think about real situations.

Discussion

In summary we note some of the issues to which respondents drew our attention.

It was clear that on the various occasions on which information is exchanged there are at least two, and probably more, people involved. Each has their own agenda and set of objectives for the meeting or visit but the interchange can easily be dominated by the person most used to the situation. In the complex and emotional period of selecting or entering a residential establishment it is the home manager and staff who are the seasoned campaigners and their interests—however benign and focused on the resident—will tend to prevail. *Home Truths* goes some way to demonstrating how the information needs of residents and their carers can be met but falls somewhere short of challenging traditional approaches and prompting creative thought about how to ensure the elderly people themselves have time and continuing opportunities to express their views.

The Way Forward

The guidelines were universally welcomed and there is a clear need for guidance in this area.

One aspect which was highlighted was a need to clarify that information is not only about written materials or details provided as part of a particular procedure or meeting. As *Home Truths* endorses, homes do need to provide written information about the services they run and in the kind of detail that helps people to understand what is on offer. But this results in a list of facts—about facilities and meal times, for example—that can be easily checked or demonstrated and from which all homes sound very much the same. Much more difficult is the crucial information about what an establishment feels like to live in—how people treat and respect each other and the ambience of the place. This too is information and the kind which most concerns people. Managers and their staff need to think about how best to provide opportunities for people to get a sense of these important aspects.

Potential residents, their relatives or advocates also need time and help to prepare for the processes of selecting or entering a home. There is room, on the evidence of our interviews, for people to take a much more robust stance—in the sense of preparing questions, checking, going back and asking more questions, asking if something can be done differently, making demands. The elderly person, however frail and however much in crisis, still has the right to be an active and questioning customer or the right to have someone to act for them.

A guide to good practice in this area might, thus, need to address not only the practice and procedures of service providers but also the rights and responsibilities of users and practical ways of exercising these.

In developing guidelines for information exchange many of our respondents advocated the kind of approach which outlines the purposes and tasks, helps to clarify whose interests are involved, alerts people to potentially difficult or sensitive areas and provides advice on how practice guides and materials can be produced which are relevant for the individual home.

We know from other projects in CHI how important it has been for local staff to have a sense of ownership and a stake in practice and training developments. Similarly, deciding on how to provide good information and in sensitive and timely ways could be a shared undertaking. Managers and staff could be guided in working together with current residents and their relatives to develop their own information policy and practice and range of materials, contacts and networks.

Information and Choice

Looking at both pieces of work—one addressing the macro-level the other micro-level issues of information provision and exchange—highlights some important points for the development of networks and providing information for service users. The Programme has helped to demonstrate the importance of information but the work has also raised questions about the way information is provided and used for different purposes by different people.

One of the underlying issues is that information—in whatever form—is a way of communicating thoughts and ideas, opinion as well as facts, hard as well as soft data. It is an instrument—a means to an end, not an end in itself. There were strong indications that most people—managers, staff, residents and relatives—need help in assessing the origins, purposes, authority, accuracy and relevance of the information they receive on the one hand, and how to use it on the other. Information is never neutral: it has to be interpreted in order to be used appropriately. Within and across care service organisations there are different priorities and interests. At the level of the care home we have seen the importance of recognising and involving the various groupings with an interest in how the home is run. At the institutional level, too, there are issues about access to knowledge and the link between knowledge and power.

The origins of the Programme's work in the Wagner review linked information provision with the promotion of choice. Information produced by service agencies is unlikely, on its own, to empower users or increase choice. Such provision is service-led and likely to be prepared and disseminated by people strongly identified with service interests. To make an effective selection between alternatives people require systematic and comprehensive information and access to the knowledge, the opinions, experience and expertise of people 'in the know'. This implies collaboration and a pooling of knowledge between institutions, agencies and interests that currently have little experience of working together. What the PSI has done is to identify the kind of work involved in addressing information provision by SSDs and to prompt thinking about the role that this plays in providing services. What is needed next is a more integrated understanding of the information needs of, and the relationship between, service providers, purchasers and users and those who are concerned with quality assurance and control.

Chapter 5

WINDOW IN HOMES: LINKS BETWEEN RESIDENTIAL HOMES AND THE COMMUNITY

The Wagner review took the view that residential establishments should be seen as part of the community in which they are located:

> 'It should not be necessary to speak in terms of links with the community—residential establishments should so clearly be a part of the community they exist to serve' (p.51).

> (Wagner, 1988)

However, evidence to the review included commentary on the isolation of many care homes and drew attention to the kind of difficulties this can generate. Where homes are cut off it is likely that residents will not be able to use the full range of services and opportunities available in the locality. The more geographically or socially isolated the home the fewer visitors it is likely to have and, in this situation, the more likely it is that restrictive regimes and bad care practice will not be noticed or challenged. On the positive side, the development of links between the home and its local community can help to ensure that residents retain their rights as citizens through, for example, exercising choice, being actively involved in local activities and using community facilities.

The Social Care Association (Education) was commissioned to develop a better understanding of the ways in which care homes and their local communities interact and to try out ways of promoting links.

The aims of the Programme were:

- to promote more contact between residential establishments and local communities;

- to stimulate more involvement by residents in the life of the home and in outside activity;

- to create more feedback on standards of care.

As with all CHI work the aim was to consider these issues across the care groupings and sectors of provision.

The Challenge

The task was a complex one. In looking at the links and relationships between homes and their community, the researchers were asked to tackle a relatively new set of ideas and, as yet, ill-defined aspects of residential care practice and development. There were few, if any, existing frames of reference or previous studies on which the work could be based. Notions of linkage between an institution and its environment were not new but traditionally they have been seen as places apart (Miller & Gwynne 1972), often located away from town centres, cut off from the main social and commercial 'shipping routes' and out of sight.

The idea that care homes should be seen both as part of the community in which they are located and as an essential part of community care services is generally accepted in principle. However, policy guidance and practice arrangements continue to make a sharp differentiation between residential services on the one hand and services in the community on the other. The possibilities of a care home providing for a range of users—not only people in residence—and, in turn, using services available in the community, are beginning to be explored but the Window in Homes Programme faced the situation where most people were thinking of residential establishments as places apart.

The dominant model of residential care has been that of total and long term care where the person entering an establishment expects to stay throughout their life. The internal world of the residential community was expected to provide all that was needed for a fulfilled life. This notion is being increasingly challenged, especially by those working for and with people with learning disabilities. The principles of normalisation, for example, are helping to dismantle such models of total care and to replace them with integrated approaches which expect and enable people to use the mainstream services and facilities that are available to all in the community (Ramon, 1991; King's Fund, 1980).

Although community links are now generally accepted as desirable, the assumptions made about why and for whose benefit have not been systematically explored. One of the tasks for the Programme, therefore, was to establish some working definitions and to identify issues which the research should cover.

The policy climate, as we have noted, meant that the work coincided with heightening concern among all care providers, but particularly those in the independent sector, about the future shape of services, about survival and about funding. Across the Initiative we noted that managers and proprietors were increasingly aware of the importance of relationships with the local community in establishing a good reputation. Financial pressures on residential care agencies have led towards diversification on the one hand and specialisation on the other as homes seek to establish an identity and a viable niche in the market. This self-consciousness was also increased by a series of scandals during the research period—particularly in child care establishments. This image awareness was not new in that the independent sector has always had to meet the demands of external monitoring and appraisal. What was, perhaps, different was a greater awareness of users' views and their significance in terms of local networks and knowledge in building a quality image. A challenge for the Programme was to discover if there were tensions between promoting community links that enhance the image and viability of the home, on the one hand, and serving the interests of residents on the other.

How the Work was Developed

The development work covered all the care groups and sectors. The nature and resources of the Programme meant that the number of homes and agencies involved was limited. It was necessary for the researchers to explore current practice in a relatively new area of thinking in order to formulate overall guidance. The time scale involved meant that it was not, in the event, possible for the Programme to set up full-scale demonstration projects. The Programme convened an advisory group to support and provide independent comment on the work.

Literature review

Initial groundwork for the Programme took the form of a review of relevant literature (Elkan and Kelly 1991). This showed that existing literature tended to be either descriptive or simply prescriptive, with little analytical or critical work in either case. From this work the Programme adopted a working definition of 'community' which reflected common ideas about what community means:

> 'the mix of formal and informal links which make up the network of relationships between the residents who live in an establishment and those outside.'

(SCA, 1992a–e)

This definition reflects the twofold nature of community: personal relationships and links based on locality or other form of association. These may overlap, but an important distinction is that personal networks are often dispersed and reach back in time. The Programme also recognised the existence of 'an internal community' —the ties and relationships operating within the residential establishment.

Project work

Unlike other Programmes the SCA team had first to obtain ideas and information about what was going on and what constituted good practice in this area. Early work was designed to learn about current trends and to find out about ways of promoting links and relationships. Generally, the work was more concerned with exploring practice than with setting up action research projects. Overall, forty-seven establishments were involved, including all the care groups although most provided for people with learning disabilities and for elders (Appendix 4.4.3).

Work commenced with two pilot projects, each involving five establishments, which looked generally at community links and at the role of Community Service Volunteers. Building on these a series of projects were set up covering the following:

- using volunteers to enhance community links;

- residential establishments as a resource for the community;

- supporting and maintaining links when entering and leaving care establishments;

- increasing individuals' social contacts and use of community facilities;

- residents' and or voluntary committees;

- the role of communication.

Each project had its own aims, style and level of engagement or activity—many were focused on information gathering—but the following stages applied to all:

(a) Identifying possible sites and points of interest to pursue;

(b) Negotiating access, agreeing general aims and where appropriate, more detailed plans;

(c) Preparatory work carrying out an audit of the current work of the establishment;

(d) Active work with the establishment;

(e) Review, withdrawal, writing up project reports.

The aims of participant homes
Potential care homes and agencies were identified by the SCA team using existing networks and contacts. The aims of the individual homes usually centred on specific aspects of the running of the establishment: their interest in community links could not always be separated from these issues. However, there was considerable support for the idea of promoting links with local communities. It caught people's imagination, sparked off

91

discussion in staff groups and gave permission for people to think in rather different ways even where the scope for making changes or shifting attitudes was limited.

Recruiting participant homes through existing contacts was helpful in allowing the Programme to explore current practices in collaboration with care homes. However, it meant that there was no opportunity to investigate the issues in homes which were more resistant to new thinking or to opening up links. Establishments which were particularly isolated or struggling with basic problems around staffing and management might be less likely to take an interest in development but might be the very establishments which would benefit most from external community links.

However, the Programme was able to consider how to deal with difficulties. There were homes involved in the projects which had experienced serious problems. Several, for example, were concerned about their poor public image and welcomed the opportunity to look at ways of changing this.

A number of homes looked at the role of volunteers: the aims were to find ways of using volunteers to enhance social activity or to facilitate self-advocacy. This included befriending schemes, providing social activities and supporting residents' activities outside the establishment.

Other establishments focused on the connection between current residents and past or future service users. In many cases the route to doing this had been through providing resources to the local community, such as lunch clubs, use of the establishment's facilities or outreach support to former residents and other local people.

The role of the consultants

Each project was initiated by a consultant appointed by SCA and it was usually they who identified and contacted potential participants. They did not provide direct input such as offering training or selecting volunteers nor did they take a lead in setting up or running activities. Their brief was to support and review progress and join in discussions with staff and residents so that establishments developed ideas without a high level of external support. They were primarily catalysts and enablers. In all cases a key person was identified within the establishment, such as a volunteer supervisor or the home manager, and it was they who took the main role in carrying the work through.

A key task for the consultants was to carry out an audit of the current work of the home by completing a schedule developed by SCA. This gathered basic information about the purposes, policies, working practices and main characteristics of the home and provided a basis for discussing what developments might be pursued. In this way consultants stimulated thinking and prompted action which might not otherwise have taken place.

The involvement of staff

Project plans were primarily negotiated with home managers. Their support was crucial but the focus of interest was often on activities which care staff could initiate or maintain. In one volunteer project, for example, supervision was provided by the deputy manager, while the unit manager took an overall supportive interest: all staff were involved to some degree in working with and supporting the volunteer. This was facilitated by clarity and agreement about the role and purpose of the volunteer and the overall aims and objectives of the unit. The pattern of project experience suggests that staffing structures and relationships, training and philosophies of care influence the ability of establishments to facilitate community links. Several projects explored how residents might be encouraged to make more use of local facilities: the role of staff in enabling such moves was an important aspect of the work. In some cases, however, the aim was to develop initiatives which were more independent of care staff roles or control, such as using volunteers or external workers to support residents' groups.

The involvement of residents

In a number of the more exploratory projects residents were not involved at all, on the basis that no active development work was planned. Although understandable, this led to the problem that consultants were not working from a consumer-centred understanding of the relevant issues.

In all projects where active work or changes were planned which might affect them directly—such as key working—residents were consulted. In a few cases this included discussing the aims of the work.

The extent to which residents were involved once the basic aims were agreed varied widely. For example, in one home, residents worked with the manager, the consultant and a volunteer. In most projects, however, residents were not directly involved in planning or discussion. Residents' needs were defined through a survey of their views about life in the home, or the consultant interviewed residents about their experience of a scheme. Usually, consultants relied on staff perceptions and definitions of residents' interests. This was an important omission, making it difficult for the Programme to explore residents' perceptions or consider the potential barriers and disadvantages of different ideas for promoting community links.

The involvement of outsiders

Given that the work concerned the relationship between the home and outside interests and facilities it was interesting to note that people from the community were not involved in many projects. The reason for this was that the commitment to create links had to come, initially, from within the establishment. On the whole, projects pursued local links by contacting other institutions or agencies—such as schools—and relatively little work concerned more personal and individual links for residents. A number of establishments were interested in greater use of community facilities, but this was often a matter of using services which do not necessarily involve significant personal contacts. However, as we will discuss later, personal links are particularly important to people living in residential establishments since many have lost family or friendship networks.

In one sense the SCA consultants were outsiders and were seen as friends from the local community in some projects. An outsider can bring different perspectives and questions to the establishment as well as confirmation or support. Many of the ideas developed did require some form of outside input, but this was often a matter of voluntary activities and efforts and making creative use of outside possibilities. In many cases, the benefit of the consultant's input did not appear to be expertise so much as the existence of an independent person able to facilitate discussion and provide feedback and support.

Aspects of Community Links Addressed by the Projects

The projects were not set up to implement a particular model. They are best seen as a linked series in which each tackled a particular set of issues from which the experience and findings would be analysed and inform a series of practice guides to be written up at the end of the Programme.

We have found it helpful to develop the following frame which makes distinctions about the nature and purpose of the links and relationships that people living in care establishments have with outsiders. An important difference is that between contacts developed or maintained for the benefit of the individual and those which serve the home as a whole. The four categories help to clarify the level at which responsibility lies for taking some form of action and to indicate who might take the lead. We also identify those whom we see as having an interest in creating and maintaining relationships between the home and outsiders. In the next section we use these distinctions as a way of presenting and discussing the work and findings of the SCA projects.

Residents' personal links and networks

Across CHI, people living in care establishments told us—or implied in what they were saying—that one of their main difficulties was that of isolation. People referred to social and emotional isolation as well as physical constraints on getting out and about.

In terms of the role and tasks of staff, this implies the need for discussion with people on an individual basis both to understand and preserve existing contacts and to help people to create networks, make friends inside and outside the home. This might include recognising the importance of past relationships as well as making new contacts.

Residents themselves, their families and carers can be active and take responsibility for ensuring that such relationships are established or maintained. However, this means overcoming the various restraints they experience through institutional living and other barriers such as stigma.

Several projects focused on such issues:

- supporting the setting up of a befriending scheme in a voluntary home for people with learning difficulties;

- a review of admission procedures in an SSD elderly people's home;

- an oral history project with a local school in an SSD elderly people's home;

- looking at ways of involving local people through voluntary and social links in an SSD home for elders;

- looking at a scheme for helping formerly homeless men to establish ordinary links.

Residents' use of local facilities and opportunities

The benefit of questioning established patterns of using—or not using—outside facilities was apparent to us across the care groups. Staff and residents easily fall into an acceptance of what is or is not possible which is more often defined by traditional notions of what people want or are able to do than real life aspirations and capabilities.

Equally, there are all sorts of ways that people can contribute to the life of the community and have a voice in what is provided and how things are run. These may be very individual arrangements or made for the residents on a more collective basis.

Supporting people through the transition from residential care to more independent living also requires knowledge about what is available in the community and understanding the continuing links that the individual might need with staff and friends in the home.

These possibilities imply outreach work from the home and discussions by staff and residents with, for example, local clubs and leisure centres, political organisations, campaign groups, day centres, sports facilities, churches, housing associations, colleges, job centres.

Projects included:

- recruiting volunteers to extend the range of activities for people with learning difficulties and for people with sensory impairments;

- work on policy around risk taking as a means for staff to facilitate community links for people with learning difficulties;

- looking at support for young people leaving care in two SSD children's homes: a large establishment with a specific leaving care unit and a small home providing outreach support for leavers.

The home as a whole: its relationship with friends, neighbours, outside bodies and agencies

Across CHI, care home managers and proprietors were concerned about the way their establishment was regarded in the wider community. Particularly for those running homes for elders this concern was fuelled by anxieties about attracting customers and survival. In homes for young people and for people with disabilities, the concern was about preserving the rights of and opportunities for the resident. There were many examples throughout CHI of the stigmatisation and discrimination that care homes and their residents can face from local people. Such problems imply a role for leadership: the task of representing the establishment as a whole is one for management but here too, there is a role for residents and frontline staff.

The home as a whole may be a resource for individuals and groups from the community. There are potential conflicts here between the interests of residents and those who use the home for other reasons but the notion of the care home as a resource centre is well established.

Projects exploring such issues included:

• work to promote positive local links for a number of homes with a poor or stigmatised local reputation. These included an establishment for young people and a therapeutic facility for people with drug and alcohol problems where links with past community were seen as a problem;

• helping to build a positive reputation for a home following a major incident of malpractice;

• supporting staff of an SSD run home in developing a lunch club to encourage links with local black elders in a multi-ethnic inner city community;

• work of a private home in providing support services to local elders;

• plans for an SSD 'linked service centre' for elders;

• plans for reusing resources of an SSD home for people with physical disabilities to cater for other people with disabilities living in the area;

• looking at two dispersed residential schemes for people with learning disabilities.

Internal relationships

One of the aspects of life in residential establishments which both the SCA and CESSA researchers considered was that of internal relationships. The culture and climate of an establishment is a reflection of the way people regard and respect each other—as colleagues and as fellow residents. Creating a climate of openness and trust in which people feel that they belong, feel secure and free to participate fully is a management responsibility but not that of management alone. The work of IQA shows how residents can share in reviewing life and work in the home.

The Programme anticipated that good internal relationships might well be the basis for good communication and relationships with outsiders.

Projects focusing on these issues included:

- exploring the roles of volunteers or external workers in supporting residents' committees or self advocacy groups in two homes for people with learning difficulties;

- looking at the role of voluntary committees in a voluntary home for elders;

- enhancing communication within the home, including the use of keyworkers.

Learning from the Projects

What does the experience of the projects tell us about the nature and purpose of links? What are the needs of different care groups? How may links best be pursued and what helps or hinders the process? What are the resource and cost implications?

The Nature and Purpose of Links

Following our earlier frame we look first at personal links and networks, using mainstream facilities, the home as a community resource and at internal relationships. We also comment on two further issues which the projects explored: the roles of volunteers and the concerns of black and ethnic minority groups.

Personal links and networks

The work of the projects confirmed that the quality of someone's lifestyle across all the care groups is intimately connected with their personal relationships and feeling connected to their families and other social networks.

Some homes already had several volunteers befriending individual residents. Although such relationships started up in a somewhat formal way, those which worked well became more personal and enduring. However, the project which aimed to set up a befriending scheme came up against the problem that there was no easy way of recruiting a pool of people with the time and interest to make links. The role of relatives was not considered directly in this context but the kind of experience that families and relatives have, now being articulated by the Relatives Association, suggests that these important relationships are not fully appreciated by care establishments.

A project which looked at admissions procedures recognised that this was a critical experience and a time when the exchange of information about the resident and their lifestyle, their needs and expectations, could help staff to understand their important links and relationships. In the event this exercise was limited and the checklist for staff which resulted was more concerned with ensuring that physical needs were understood and could be met. This in many ways echoes the work of PSI (Dawson et al, 1992) in which the information exchange around the point of admission tended to focus more on physical and medical issues than exploring the history, the social and personal links of the potential resident. This may say something about the traditional patterns which service providers have built up and which are hard to recast in a more user-centred mode.

Some projects were looking at rather different issues relating to protection and control. Preserving the relationships and social networks of drug abusers, for example, might be problematic. Nonetheless, the establishment for people with drug problems was broadly successful in developing alternative social networks and links in the neighbourhood. Equally, where children have been placed away from troubled families, continuing links needed careful handling.

Where establishments have a regional or a national catchment area the problems of maintaining contacts, or even of knowing what the local community should be, are more severe. Children may be uprooted from every meaningful link, only to find that attempts to make links in the area of a large establishment are considered a problem. Children in one establishment, for example, were cut off from their original area and felt they didn't belong, yet they were discouraged from settling or making links in the locality, partly due to fears of creating some sort of ghetto. Even in establishments for elders, where such problems should not apply, residents' links with kin are easily undermined. Relatives feelings about continuing contact may be affected by unresolved guilt about the move, coupled with uncertainty about how they can continue a close, caring relationship.

One problem, perhaps, lies in assuming that links depend on outsiders visiting the home. However, social opportunities are often based on activities outside the home, including the workplace, and that is why access to a range of local facilities and opportunities was seen as important.

Links with mainstream facilities and outside contacts

Project experience endorsed that access to local facilities was highly valued by residents. Many residents did not want to use specialised day care services which were segregated and which did not generally provide socially valued roles. Some residents wanted to move on to real jobs rather than continue work in day centres which was low paid and uninteresting. They recognised that taking part in leisure or other classes would not necessarily lead to social or other contacts but could be a step towards this.

Although several projects focused on the use of ordinary facilities rather than specialised or segregated ones, we noted that many took a rather limited view of what this meant—tending to see the possibilities in rather institutional terms, like attending the day centre, visiting the doctor, attending college. Where a home is supporting a move to more independent living, the implications for care staff are clearly more wide-ranging than that.

Projects highlighted some of the barriers which made it difficult for people to move out and about. Some of these were obvious and frequently concerned lack of suitable transport. However, the underlying issues about residents being able and enabled to use ordinary facilities and make relationships in the community related rather to the culture of the home and the assumptions made about the level of care needed by residents. One such issue, recognised in several projects, was that of risk taking. Staff in many homes across the CHI were anxious about the vulnerability of their residents. They were concerned in case people were taken advantage of, behaved in a way that would bring criticism on the home, got into physical danger or got confused or lost. One agency began to tackle this when staff asked for a policy: they wanted a clear understanding about their level of responsibility if people with learning disabilities went out on their own and got into any sort of trouble.

Another issue was the extent to which residents themselves were able to take the initiative. Their ability or willingness to do so was linked partly with age and mobility and partly with the level of independence expected or allowed by the particular establishment. Personal expectations vary with experience and it was often establishments which were open in their outlook and encouraging towards residents that were able to take up opportunities and question any barriers experienced.

The home as a whole: its relationships with the community
The projects revealed a number of different issues about the way a home was regarded in the locality and several projects looked at how they might improve the general image. Some were concerned with extending the role of the care home by providing extra services to the local community: others were looking at the benefit of reciprocal relationships.

Several projects looked at the diversification of residential establishments into resource centres, for example, day care, respite care and other services. One agency had planned the diversification of a home to a resource centre without consultation with the existing residents: the lack of appreciation of their interests was underlined when they were not invited to the opening event. This kind of example indicates how commercial and other pressures can impinge markedly on people in residential care. However, the projects did not explore the impact on residents or their local community nor point up particular issues and tensions that might have arisen and how staff dealt with them.

There are other, less formal ways, in which residential care establishments may be a resource and these were explored in other projects. For example, a children's establishment continued to provide support for young people after they had left care. The home was a small one and young people were able to settle nearby so that their relationships with each other and with staff could be maintained. This was an interesting example where the young adults had the support of, in effect, a kinship-type network and were not expected to move into more independent living without support.

The projects also explored some interesting situations where residents were able to do voluntary work in the neighbourhood. An establishment for adults recovering from drug problems promoted the potential benefit of community links both for their residents and for local people. The residents valued these contacts. Indeed, one resident continued her voluntary work with a frail elderly person beyond the planned period and she felt the experience had changed her image of herself in a positive way. Another found that his work at a drop-in centre for people with mental health problems helped him to reflect on his past and to develop self confidence. Another example involved a link between a home for elders and a school in an oral history project which the staff felt was valued and beneficial both to residents and the children involved. It was clear from such projects that part of the value was in providing the opportunity for residents to experience themselves in a different way and to be valued.

The image of the home as a whole was one which was tackled by a home for children and young people which had had a poor reputation for some time. Neighbours and people in the immediate locale can often be highly anxious and critical of people whom they see as being in any way deviant. In this project staff took an active role in talking to local groups, talking to the media and, perhaps the most important of all, agreeing a policy within their agency about how to respond to external complaints and criticisms. Residents were also involved through open days and voluntary activities in the neighbourhood. Their involvement helped to dispel misconceptions about the young people and offered more constructive ways of coming into contact with local people.

Internal relationships
Several projects looked at the quality of communication within the home and how residents might be helped to participate more. A key project here involved volunteers working with a self-advocacy group of people with learning difficulties. This involved quite intensive work over a period of

time, gradually helping people to express their questions, ideas and views. In many ways this kind of work links with that of the IQA projects which were also concerned with helping people to speak out.

Other projects looked at ways of supporting residents' committees but clarity about the purpose of these groups was important. There is a great deal of difference between self-advocacy groups and those which are focused on social activities or providing a chance for discussion. None of the committees involved had a role or direct voice in the management of the establishment. Volunteers played important roles as facilitators but the use of advocates was not explored. Some establishments were managed by voluntary committees but these did not involve residents directly.

Another area of work looked at internal relationships between staff and residents and the role of keyworking. Although this is accepted as good residential practice many establishments do not have such arrangements and smaller homes often prefer informal approaches. However, effective keyworking depends on good existing relationships between staff and an understanding and acceptance of its purpose among staff and residents. Residents, in particular, need to be involved and to have a say in the allocation of keyworkers.

Black perspectives and equality issues

Two projects focused on the experience of people from ethnic minority groups. Both involved social services run homes for elders in inner city areas. Both had a number of black staff but few black residents. In most other establishments across the Programme there were few or no black residents and consultants did not focus on these issues partly because staff did not see their relevance. However, black residents are often in situations of extreme isolation in establishments which are unable to welcome or respond to their cultural needs or expectations.

In one inner city establishment, staff identified the lack of black residents as an issue to be tackled. They hoped that starting a drop-in for local black elders would alter this balance, provide some contacts for the two black residents and change the image of the home with black people in the area. A great deal of work was done and, although only a few people came to the drop-in, staff felt the group had benefited one black resident in particular. This work was also an opportunity for black workers in the home to take the lead and for the establishment to recognise and gain from their interest and experience.

In another project, which did not focus on ethnicity or equality issues, race emerged as a significant issue for the one black resident. His experience of a therapeutic community type regime had helped him in thinking about the past, his own needs and problems, and the importance of ethnic identity. However, he felt the (predominantly white) institution was only able to help him resolve these problems in a limited way. His experience highlighted the particular significance of links for black people and the problems of maintaining identity in white institutions. It illustrates how race and culture was an issue for all establishments: how far does a home convey an atmosphere in which all can feel a clear and positive sense of identity?

Using volunteers to enhance community links

The Wagner review raised questions about the role of volunteers in promoting choice and a sense of integration. These were explored further in the literature review (Elkan and Kelly, 1991) and in a number of projects. The general lesson was that volunteers may fulfil roles which staff cannot and that volunteering is most effective when viewed as complementary to staff roles and is properly planned and supported.

Project experience suggested the following basic guidelines:

- clear definition of volunteer's role and the purpose of their involvment. This should be discussed with users and care workers;

- volunteers should be seen as working to meet residents' interests: fulfilling their own objectives or meeting their own needs are secondary;

- structured but relevant and flexible arrangements are required for the recruitment and selection of volunteers;

- volunteers require adequate information about the establishment, its purposes and philosophy and how their role fits in;

- they require induction and supervision, support and appropriate training;

- planned review, change over time and withdrawal.

Volunteers' roles focused on how residents can engage in outside activities and contribute more actively to the life of the home, including feedback on standards of care. Although workers, volunteers and users expressed positive views, their comments suggested there is a point beyond which residential services, no matter how open their approach, cannot pursue community integration. This is particularly so when care groups experience stigma. Volunteers can contribute to better links within and outside the home, but likewise, what they can achieve is limited. Perhaps the greatest prospect for change is in the potential role of volunteers in encouraging users to speak up and speak out for themselves.

One project using Community Service Volunteers provided a useful example since it's brief was to enhance activities outside the establishment and self advocacy within it. Feedback from all project participants confirmed that the project was successful in terms of its own objectives. The residents were able to be involved in more leisure activity in non-segregated facilities. They enjoyed and valued this. However, this did not make them feel more a part of their local community or more accepted by neighbours. They felt more fundamental changes were necessary to bring about a real sense of belonging. Similarly, they gained confidence and 'spoke up' but they remained cautious about what a self-advocacy group can achieve.

Positive indicators from volunteer projects included:

- residents talking about the value of the volunteer placement to them;

- residents going out more, pursuing new interests;

- residents gaining in confidence and voice;

- volunteers' own learning and enjoyment;

- enthusiasm for continuing the work after SCA's withdrawal;

- raised staff awareness of residents' social needs.

But there were also indicators for caution including residents' awareness of:

- the limitations of what a volunteer can do and be;

- the limits of self-advocacy when long-term and basic changes are desired;

- the persistence of prejudice or stigma;

- resource and other constraints on continuing an initiative which they feel can be beneficial for them.

The Needs of Different Care Groups
Project work was carried out in homes for all the care groups although most work was done in relation to elders and people with learning disabilities. The different groups highlighted some different needs in relation to links and connections with the community although most issues were common to all.

Children
Key issues here related to a child's removal from previous ties, including kin and in some cases their local community, school, friends, clubs and so

on. The time-limited nature of care means that a major challenge for the children is in moving towards an independent adult life, with ordinary and reliable social ties and means of practical, social and emotional support.

Young people have many bases for ties—such as school—but usually experience stigma in the locality of residential care homes. Leaving care is a particularly difficult period of transition for young people who have lived in institutional settings and who generally lack family support. Staff as well as young adults needed opportunities to discuss their anxieties and to develop skills in outreach work. Making links to support positive contacts in the local community is time-consuming and may work best where the home continues to be available to the young adult.

Adults with disabilities

We have noted that people with disabilities experienced particular problems around access or communication, linked to poor access and arrangements for disabilities in many community facilities. Residents also reported a major problem of isolation and stigma, often based on ignorance and assumptions which were not helped by living in relatively isolated care homes. Personal links were deeply affected by individuals' careers as service users through moving from one institution to another, or the view that past networks are part of the problem to be overcome.

Overcoming isolation and stigmatisation was an important aspect of promoting more understanding and connection with the local community and particularly so for care homes that have traditionally been seen as places apart.

Elders

Although elders do not suffer the forms of stigma shared, to some degree, by all other care groups, they are frequently isolated from personal or local networks. There is a tendency to assume dependency and that residential care is a permanent option. Such attitudes and lack of mobility tended to work against maintaining community links, including those with relatives. Additionally, the move into residential care was often seen as a last resort and associated with guilt or shame. As a result of such feelings, relatives and friends need help to establish the degree of involvement they wish.

What Helps and Hinders the Promotion of Links?

We look now at the kind of conditions that promoted outreach and the building of relationships and at aspects of practice that helped or hindered links with the community.

Size, character and location

There was nothing in the project experience to suggest that size was a determining factor, but larger establishments appeared to have more problems with community integration. While small homes were less likely to encounter stigma, residents could still suffer from isolation without proactive work and encouragement from staff or volunteers. Design and appearance mattered as well as size, because of the image of the establishment which was portrayed. An ordinary but well cared for home was more likely to convey a normal positive image for its residents. Many homes were in large, if beautiful grounds, miles from shops, cut off from transport routes. Geographical isolation of this sort is particularly difficult to overcome: the apparent advantages of a calm and pleasant environment can prevent staff from appreciating the problems of isolation and dislocation for residents.

History and reputation

Some establishments had suffered from being located on sites with a history of institutional services, thus creating barriers to be overcome. But projects showed that there is much that establishments can do to overcome negative reputations and images. On the whole, they confirm evidence from elsewhere (e.g. hospital closure studies) that a proactive approach, which incorporates informing and educating local people, is more effective than keeping a low profile. The latter may be effective in avoiding stigma but it is then more difficult for active work on establishing links to take place. Past experiences help to form the prevailing culture of the home and also influence the attitudes of staff, their perceptions of residents and their confidence in making links.

Organisational factors

Organisational factors had an important influence on the chances of any innovation being pursued or proving effective. For example, where management and staffing systems were not clear and adequate, establishments were preoccupied with resolving internal matters.

There was some indication that many home managers in larger organisations felt constrained in their freedom to initiate links with the community. Many were uncertain if they had the authority or permission to represent the home to other service agencies, to social organisations or local community and interest groups. This was an issue which emerged across CHI: there were many examples where there seemed to be some lack of clarity between the home manager and senior staff about who takes responsibility. When this relates to the outside image and reputation of the home, social services departments, for example, have tended to be defensive and home managers have had little freedom to speak directly to people in the community. At the other end of the scale owner-managers are in a position of representing their interests very directly but they can lack time and resources to make links into local networks and are not necessarily concerned with enhancing links for residents.

Management committees

Several projects looked at the roles of management and other committees. A number of homes had voluntary management committees and several had committees to organise social and leisure activities. However, it should not be assumed that voluntary committees constitute community links for residents or that they are more democratic or integrated than other forms of management. Where establishments had residents' committees or self-advocacy groups these did not have significant power or influence. Several projects were able to show how the independence and effectiveness of residents' committees could be enhanced by using outside facilitators—other professionals or volunteers—but this did not guarantee empower-ment for residents. None of the projects explored the role of individual advocacy or wider citizen advocacy schemes. In none of the establish-ments did residents have a strong voice in management, although most were working towards enabling resident involvement in some way. One self-advocacy group, for example, was able to request a change in the time of staff meetings so that they could send two representatives. In contrast, another was more of a discussion group with no definable advocacy role or link with decision making and management.

The roles of staff, managers and agencies
It was important for the Programme to consider whether the ideas or activities initiated would have been tackled without the facilitating role of the consultant. The examples of community links across the projects showed that there were many innovations taking shape, but often these were unrecognised and unsupported by the agencies.

Achievements came about because the specific efforts of staff and volunteers were sustained by internal supports. Home managers played a key role in enabling or hindering such efforts. The best results came when roles and philosophies were clear and where managers had the confidence and ability to delegate or share responsibility with other staff, residents and outsiders.

The main issue here was how far people—managers, staff or residents—could take the initiative in defining desirable links and finding ways to promote them. The problem often seemed to stem from a lack of awareness or imagination: once ideas were flowing, commitment was secured and practical issues were less difficult to overcome. The consult-ants provided a stimulus, focused attention on external links and in many cases, it was clear that without them little might have happened. It seemed that some kind of external stimulus was helpful—perhaps essential in many homes.

Resource and cost implications
The costs and effort involved in project work varied. The main costs were in staff time. Few projects required material resources, equipment or extra paid help. Activities, in most cases, were on a limited scale and were managed within ordinary working routines: such work was not generally regarded as having a measurable cost. Homes unable to free time and

mobilise the commitment and interest of staff would, therefore, be less likely to manage.

In most cases a far longer time was needed to get started than the six months that consultants had anticipated. This suggests that establishments paced the work to some extent according to what they could manage and tells something about the scope and pace of work which is feasible in care establishments.

The most costly projects were those using full-time volunteers. Costs related to providing good supports for the volunteers which included time devoted to preparation and selection, supervision and training. Additionally, volunteers providing more intensive input needed expenses, allowances and in some cases, accommodation.

In one project, for example, time spent in recruitment and selection were provided by CSV and were not a cost to the establishment, but the information for recruitment was prepared by staff with assistance from CSV and SCA. The volunteers received weekly 'pocket money' and were provided with rented accommodation off site. The key cost in staff time was for weekly (or fortnightly) supervisions with a senior care worker. Staff involved felt there were no additional time costs as support was fitted with everyday work without problems. Additionally, a training day was organised with an external trainer. This day was used for the benefit of staff, volunteer and residents, who all participated.

Against the costs or efforts involved in the placement, staff felt strongly that the project had been beneficial and had placed few burdens on their time. This was assisted, in their view, by having a good volunteer who worked well with staff and residents. However, the costs of the trainer and the volunteer were covered by SCA in this case. Although it was agreed by residents and staff that the project should continue with another placement, this was prevented by lack of money.

This project showed that even quite intensive volunteer support can offer good value for money, but that this cannot be achieved without some costs. It also highlighted the experience of other projects—that there is not a large pool of untapped time and effort around, waiting to be used. Good volunteers may be hard to find. In another project, an existing volunteer took on the role of volunteer co-ordinator. She was in an excellent position to contact local people who might offer some time and possibly share a mutual interest, such as sports, with a resident.

It must be borne in mind that using volunteers has cost implications. Adequate planning, supervision and support are vital to using volunteers well and for residents' benefit. Much of this work can be a part of everyday activity but this is only likely to occur in establishments with an adequate staff structure and existing budgets for training and supporting workers properly. This is not always the case.

Project Outcomes

The majority of Window in Homes projects were concerned with exploring and learning about practice which supports community links. A smaller number of projects aimed for development through changes in policies, practices or attitudes of workers and other people. One of the main lessons was that shifts of this sort—involving basic assumptions and attitudes—require thought and development over a long period. In many cases the ideas contributed to a radical change in ethos in the establishment.

Benefits for Homes

Although consultants completed a form of audit to obtain information about the home this was not used explicitly to define the project work and relate it to the overall work of the home. As a result, the work on community links was often seen as an additional and optional activity rather than fundamentally connected to the quality of service provided overall.

We found limited evidence of impact in the homes—on policies, practices or workers' attitudes. Where aims for development in the home (e.g. introducing a keyworker system) were not achieved this was often due to underlying staffing or management issues which needed attention before the work could progress. In most cases, a longer time run would have been required to see significant changes take place. The main achievements stemmed from particular initiatives, such as running a drop-in club or using volunteers to facilitate a more independent residents' group. These were ideas the establishments had planned themselves but the intervention of the Programme had helped them to move forward, perhaps faster than they might otherwise have done. A key problem here was that residents themselves were not often involved in the plans although they had usually been consulted once ideas had been formed.

Staff Attitudes

Consultants recognised that staff approval and some measure of involvement was important for enabling and sustaining change. Even where care staff were not actively involved, their views were generally positive and interested. However, problems with staff support and communication meant that certain projects did not achieve their own objectives. In such cases, attention needed to be given more directly to staff requirements before wider objectives could be met.

Where workers and residents were actively involved—for example, in communicating a realistic image of the establishment in the local area and media—this helped them to feel positive about themselves and positive about the identity of the home. Generally the projects stimulated discussion and an awareness amongst staff that things can change, can be questioned, can be improved.

Benefits for Agencies

The projects did not set out to work at a strategic level. However, if good practices and positive links are to be sustained then the support of the agency is vital. In certain establishments, motivation for involvement with the research was a lack of support from their own agency. In private establishments a related issue was how to form and use networks for support and ideas.

In a climate of change and uncertainty, a positive initiative on community links may be seen as valuable but fail to figure highly enough in the order of priorities. For example, one volunteer project, despite very positive reports from staff and residents, failed to secure modest funding to continue the project and although other unit managers were aware of the project, the ideas were not picked up elsewhere.

Benefits for Residents

Not all projects involved residents in activities or in commenting on the ideas being explored. This meant that consultants did not fully explore the implications of existing or new practices for residents' quality of life and projects were not informed by residents' views.

We noted, however, some significant benefits for residents. In an oral history project, for example, staff saw residents as more alert and responsive. Where a full-time volunteer had been supporting a self-advocacy group, residents were enthusiastic about the benefits, although they saw the limits as well. Their views were supported by staff comments about their growth in confidence and ability to speak up.

It does appear that planned and sensitive use of volunteers may have greater potential for residents' lives than staff-led initiatives. Volunteers may not provide a bridge to the community as such but can offer more ordinary, independent and valued opportunities and options. Volunteers are in a good position to support initiatives—such as residents' committees—where independence from staff is important. Going out and doing things with a volunteer is a different experience from going out with staff, not only because individual activities become more feasible but because the relationship is different. Individual relationships with volunteers may form a first step towards friendship, in that relationship or with others outside the service. However, the project which aimed to set up a befriending scheme found that there is not necessarily a large pool of people with the time and interest available for this.

Since few projects focused on individual links it was not surprising that we found little evidence of enhanced personal relationships for residents. Generally, encouraging family contacts is considered an integral aspect of good residential care practice, yet it is still an area that is often neglected. A review of admission procedures in one project might have been an opportunity to consider ways of maintaining family links but this aspect was not highlighted.

The Practice Guides

The main output of the Programme is a series of booklets (SCA, 1992a-e; SCA, 1993a & b) which are concise, accessible and practical guides to thinking through ideas about improving community links. The Guides draw on the projects and each tackles a particular theme. However, since the projects were mainly exploratory, the guides do not set out detailed advice on how to set up activities. They are useful documents for prompting discussion and thought about practice rather than describing programmes for change.

The Guides were produced at the end of the Programme and we can comment, therefore, on the extent to which they address practical issues of implementation gathered from the projects. They acknowledge and set out some of the potential barriers to good practice but do not, on the whole, explore these fully.

Widening Horizons: a general introductory guide to the issues, setting out common definitions and assumptions about community and the nature and role of residential establishments. It raises a set of questions and thinking points and looks at some aspects of resistance as well as opportunities for creating links.

Voluntary Links: a guide to involving volunteers in developing contacts between residential establishments and the wider community. It is short, clear and systematic, giving basic outlines of the questions and planning which need to be considered. It gives limited consideration to some of the problems in involving volunteers but does not distinguish between different types of volunteering, the levels and forms of preparation and support needed. Its key contribution is in setting out in clear steps the decisions, plans and stages establishments need to go through. It highlights the importance of involving residents and staff, of working out the aim and purpose of volunteer placements and of providing adequate training and support.

Positive Images: a commentary on how establishments might take a pro-active role in overcoming negative images of residents or the establishment. It suggests how to improve communication with local communities and foster good relationships. This is relevant to all homes but particularly to those affected by stigmatising public attitudes.

Giving and Taking: focuses on the use of residential establishments as resources to the local community as well as suggesting, in its title, wider considerations about the importance of two-way contact. It gives some examples of resource centres and refers to dilemmas about residents' rights and privacy. It does not take a position or give advice on this nor does it comment on the impact of such developments on residents. This is an aspect which does need to be addressed as more homes are looking at how they can diversify.

Communication Begins at Home: the general message here is that good external links need to rest on a foundation of good communication within the home. The Guide discusses the relevant issues, grounded in the project experience, using examples of the types of problems which can arise and types of practice which may enhance internal communication. This includes some key points on the running of residents' committees, on keyworking and on means of staff communication. It notes the need to consider the balance of power within establishments and the importance of communication to residents' feelings of control over decisions and events. The Guide also includes a brief section on the needs of people with communication problems, although a longer and more specialised publication would generally be needed to follow this up.

Most recently published are *Lasting Impressions*: a guide to reconsidering the image of residential establishments in their local community and *Blurring Boundaries*: a further general booklet on issues raised by considering community links.

Discussion

The Window In Homes Programme raised a number of important questions about the place of care homes in their local community and ways in which residents' lives may be more integrated socially.

In this chapter we have outlined the main types of links which appeared useful in understanding how the Programme approached its task. Here we look at some of the issues which were raised in evaluation and which deserve further thought.

The Nature of Community
The Programme took a view of community as characterised by both the locality and the personal networks of individuals. How far has it re-examined the notion of community for people in residential care?

We have noted how the idea of community is difficult to define except in a very broad way. The basic principle followed was that residential care should be a part of the community it serves. The projects explored attitudes and practice which were thought to have an impact on the social connections of the establishment and its residents. However, our discussion of project design and outcomes highlights that, in many ways, the meaning of community was assumed rather than fully discussed by those participating in the projects. Managers and care workers, for example, most usually understood questions of links and relationships outside the home to be local contacts. Many had had no cause or opportunity to consider the issues in relation to the needs and wishes of individual residents.

The main interest of individual residents—here and across CHI—was in personal relationships and social contacts. Community for them meant friends, family, wherever they might be. For others, the sense of community lay in shared values or cultural norms: for others local friends and contacts were important. We suggest that a sense of belonging comes from connection with and acceptance by those who are important to the individual and that 'community' should be defined according to individual as well as collective meanings.

The Residential Establishment as a Community?

One concept which was implicit in the design of projects was that of the internal community of the home. Residential care has to balance private and public living, individual and collective interests, by its very nature. Project experience indicated that the nature of internal relationships had implications for external links. On the whole, project aims succeeded where relationships within the home were valued and open to change, and where workers and residents felt supported by others. Projects which did not achieve their aims were affected by internal difficulties like unsupportive management, uncertainty about the future, poor morale or lack of communication between managers, staff and residents.

A small number of homes viewed themselves as therapeutic communities, with an emphasis on fostering communication and positive social relationships. However, these often focus on personal change and their philosophies, while promoting a particular form of internal community, may mask differences between groups or individuals and subtly prevent external relationships.

Across the care groups we were aware of numbers of people who viewed their life in establishments positively: they valued the company of others, gained confidence from their association with people like themselves and identified strongly with the home. For them the notion of an internal community was a real and supportive one. However, there were also many examples where residents had no sense of belonging. In many homes, for example, it is rare for residents to have a say in who enters. In larger establishments in particular it is hard for people to feel it is their home at all. Nonetheless, relationships between residents are highly important and can be enhanced through groups (whether for advocacy, management or social activity).

Networks of mutual support amongst former residents may also be particularly important for young adults and representatives from user organisations stressed that residential care which involves small, self chosen groups is most likely to be a positive choice. Such a setting may combine the advantages of collective living—company, mutual support, a sense of community—with greater opportunities for individual and personal needs and interests to be supported.

112

The Nature and Purpose of Links?

Evaluation highlighted how ideas about links may operate on two levels—institutional and personal. There is a tendency for establishments to promote institutional links, which reflect the institutional nature of residents' experience and their 'careers' in the service system. For example—between elderly people's homes and schools or between establishment and day centre. Given the context of isolation and stigma for people in care and the history of institutionalism, it remains a matter of debate whether institutional links should be seen as positive or potentially stigmatising.

Whether links between people in residential care and in other institutions are seen as positive will depend on the nature and purpose of those links. Some of these more formal links have introduced an element of reciprocity which is taken for granted in most ordinary social relationships but is highly valued. They may also provide an opportunity for staff to develop contacts with people outside the establishment. The IQA experience suggested that there are ways in which structured links with outsiders may help to promote an open outlook and more individual or personal links with local people. Such developments cannot be assumed, however, and there was evidence that establishments would have to work to create such contacts.

We commented earlier that it is the more individual and personal links which matter most. Within the establishment these might include relationships with other residents, with care staff and sometimes with other staff or volunteers. It is often the case that staff without a direct care role, such as activities organisers have stronger personal relationships with residents. Keyworking is widely regarded as good practice, in order to promote more personal relationships between care staff and residents, but it is still rare for residents to have any say in the choice of keyworker. The experience of the project which focused on this suggests that the aims of keywork will not simply be achieved by setting up a system, particularly if relationships between staff and residents are poor.

It can be questioned, however, whether keyworkers are the appropriate people to have closer relationships with the residents. Their role should, perhaps, be seen as providing support and helping to create opportunities for residents to form new relationships and find social contacts outside the home. We noticed a significant lack of imagination among workers whose thinking about the care needs of residents was confined by long established patterns, and set practices and assumptions. Promoting links and personal contacts requires open and creative thinking—care staff can be helped to become more flexible by listening to residents.

Using mainstream opportunities was often seen as a way of promoting links but the limitations of such work needed further exploration. A distinction can be drawn between community presence and community participation as aspects of ordinary living (Ramon, 1991). The nature and signficance of links will differ in each case but the former can be seen as a prerequisite to the latter. So, use of ordinary facilities such as shops or hairdressers—mentioned as links in a number of project reports—could be seen as elements of a community presence which are important but not sufficient to be considered links in themselves. Many residents recognised that more fundamental changes are needed to change their social identity and feelings of isolation or frustration. Using local facilities is valued but may not lead to development of significant social ties.

Residential Care as a Community Resource?

Although there has been interest in residential establishments as resource centres, questions remain about their impact on residents. Examples of such work were looked at in the Programme but their impact on residents, carers or the local community was not considered in detail. Are there ways of designing such bases which will not interfere with residents' private space? Or do they have little impact on what is already a compromise or confusion of public and private domains? Shifts from long-term care to a mix with short-term and respite care might also affect existing residents' privacy and personal space. If handled sensitively, the 'visitors' could provide positive links for permanent residents, but the experience of managers we interviewed is that such shifts often take place in an unplanned way, without consideration of relationships between residents. Do such developments have anything to give to residents—for example, can they improve social networks or decrease a sense of isolation? There is no clear evidence from the projects of whether this is the case and so it remains an assumption in the planning of such services.

Moves towards diversification have increased in recent years, in response to policy and legislative developments, in particular the development of care management, contracting and transfer of funding for residential services. We noted a greater interest in issues of presentation—and these were a strong theme in the projects—but they were often led by organisational and agency concerns. The shifts towards resource centres of various types need to be considered in this light. They may be founded more on concerns about institutional survival rather than concerns about the ways in which users can feel more integrated with other people and institutions in the locality. Further questions need to be raised, by those involved in residential care, about ways in which developments may be initiated and focused on the concerns and interests of existing and future service users.

The Nature of Boundaries and Barriers

How can establishments tackle the more difficult aspects of community links—such as where the client group is stigmatised or where workers feel very protective towards clients who are seen as dependent? The experience of several projects provided pointers for this, although the work was limited. One consultant focused particularly on establishments experiencing barriers of some sort, including poor reputation or legacies from the past, stigma and the need to establish better contact with ethnic minority communities. These projects have shown that there is much that can be done to overcome barriers and boundaries. Negative community attitudes are partly based on lack of accurate information, so that if contact can be increased, however slightly, positive changes are possible. This, however, requires staff time and confidence and, ideally, a high degree of resident involvement. The role of an outsider, though not essential, may be important to overcoming initial fears or resistance within an establishment and this may be achieved with the help of clear management, participative training and staff development approaches which legitimate these, for many, new tasks of outreach, negotiation and contact building.

Changes in wider social attitudes will not be achieved overnight. However, community presence is an important first step in establishing the view that people who live in residential care can and should have an ordinary and positive role to play outside the establishment. Again, if people are to be regarded as individuals rather than one of a group of service users—defined by needs and problems—there needs to be greater emphasis on enabling people to get out and about on their own terms.

Isolation and Connection
Is the Wagner connection between isolation and vulnerability to institutionalised or restrictive care valid? Reflecting on the experience of an establishment which had been the scene of a scandal, one consultant commented that a number of people crossing the threshold had not uncovered these problems. This suggests that something more than movement, or 'windows', is required. A greater degree of connection and understanding is needed alongside opportunities for staff and residents to speak out.

Living in residential care is always a compromise between the advantages (or economies) of group living and the disadvantages of lack of choice, privacy and individuality. The Programme explored how communication and structures within the home can make a difference to residents' experience and positive sense of community within the home. It has helped to highlight the importance of developing awareness and creative responses to the problems which are often found in residential care. The work of the SCA Programme has identified some of the basic issues which need to be addressed if homes, and those living and working in them, are to avoid isolation.

Chapter 6

TRAINING FOR CARE STAFF

The Wagner review and reports which have followed (eg Howe, 1992; the Warner report DOH/HMSO, 1992a) looked at the link between the quality of care service provided in care homes and staffing issues. The low morale of residential care staff has been well documented: it emerged as an important theme in evidence given to the Wagner review. The Howe report made particular reference to the relatively poor image and status of residential care as a service, both in the eyes of the public and as perceived by other professionals in the field of social care. The recommendations arising from these reports and reviews assume the following set of relationships. Low staff morale is associated as much with stress and being undervalued as it is with with low or anomalous levels of pay and long hours. Low morale leads to higher rates of sickness and staff turnover and a lack of commitment to the work.

What are these stresses? They arise partly from the nature of the work itself. In Chapter 2 we commented how, in a group-based service, staff experience pressure from working in a semi-public arena, since their practice is open to view by peers and senior colleagues. Another significant source of stress can be the emotional impact of the work. Menzies (1970) in her study of nursing showed how the

> 'close physical care of hospital patients provoked complex feelings—which included, at the professional level, fears of failure and lack of competence and at the personal level feelings of envy, anger, revulsion and problems about coping with intimacy and dependency' (Youll, 1985).

There are exact parallels in social care: staff have to find ways of coping with the considerable anxieties evoked.

Working in a team can be supportive and rewarding but there is also evidence to suggest that this, too, can be stressful. People feel a greater sense of responsibility because their actions can affect the practice of others: the team can be let down by an individual. Being accepted and keeping to the group norms are highly important to staff. Rifts and tensions in a staff group can be threatening—even persecuting—for individuals. Poor management, conflicting demands, lack of leadership will almost certainly lead to difficulties in a staff team and these, in turn, cause stress and lead to low morale.

In this way we can see how inadequate support, conflicts or inconsistencies, lack of relevant training or opportunities for staff development and team building can contribute to staff feeling undervalued, of low status and uncertain how to cope with the considerable demands of the work.

The Wagner review highlighted effective staff training and team development as an important way forward and proposed that:

'every establishment should be required to draw up a staff training plan ... (which) should be subject to inspection procedures'.

(Ch 9 Para 25, Wagner, 1988)

This report was the first to draw attention to the need for a coherent approach to staff development and training based on team working and this has been most recently endorsed by the Wagner Development Group papers (NISW/HMSO, 1993) and by recent publications on training (LGMB, 1992).

The National Institute for Social Work (NISW) was commissioned to develop training approaches and materials for basic-level care staff. The original brief from the DOH linked improving the status and morale of basic care staff with the promotion of good practice and quality care.

The brief given to the researchers was:

'to improve the quality of residential care in both the statutory and independent sectors by promoting basic training of care assistants of a kind which can readily be arranged and supervised by the managers of the homes, and will equip them with essential competencies in line with the National Vocational Qualifications framework'.

(DOH Brief 1989)

The kind of training envisaged was, therefore, locally initiated and managed opportunities for basic care workers. With the needs and resources of the small private sector home in mind, the work was targeted for care home owners and managers.

We can note, however, that the brief did not entirely embrace the Wagner recommendations nor did it assume a connection between staff support, staff development and the provision of good quality care. The focus on basic-level workers addressed a neglected area of staff training but it did not, for example, focus attention on the production of training plans, on team building or the place of development for the home as a whole.

The Context for Training Developments

Before describing and commenting on the Programme's work and its outcomes we must note some of the developments which were taking place during the life of the projects and the challenge these presented.

Community Care Implementation

As with all the CHI work, community care implementation meant that the establishments participating in this work were in the process of adapting to a new environment. The level of concern varied to some extent between public and independent sectors but there were general anxieties about funding and financial security, about contracting arrangements, about meeting inspection criteria and quality standards. The practice implications of these policy changes were significant since they required staff—especially at middle and senior management levels—to take on new work and to acquire new skills and knowledge. The agenda for training in agencies was strongly determined by these needs which fell primarily into such areas as financial management, financial and legal aspects of purchasing and contracting, assessment for services, care management and inspection.

In this climate, training for basic-level staff in residential services might have been seen as a secondary concern. However, we found that establishments across CHI considered training to be one of the most important means of promoting a quality service. The emphasis placed on the recruitment and training of qualified staff following the several scandals which occurred during the life of CHI served to endorse the importance of staffing generally and training in particular.

One of the possible trends we noted was that the identification and definition of training and staff development needs could move from the centre to provider units and from strategic to local levels. If this is so then the NISW experience of helping unit managers to define training needs in relation to their local service requirements will be of increasing relevance.

Education and Training in Social Work and NVQ

Of specific relevance to this work was the parallel development of the national system of vocational training and qualification (NVQ) based on workplace experience and the radical restructuring of education and training in social work.

NVQ is geared to enabling the individual member of staff to gain a relevant and practice-based qualification. It is a system of assessment rather than a training programme as such. One important aspect is the emphasis it places on the workplace: this has to fulfil various requirements if it is to be recognised as competent to provide experience of the necessary standard for someone to qualify. This precondition for NVQ assessment has an impact on care and practice quality.

However, we should note that the emphasis of NVQ is on how the competent workplace provides opportunities for individual workers, not the other way round.

In distinction to this, the Training for Care Staff Programme was more concerned with the contribution that the worker can make to the effective running of the care home, not only as an individual but also as a member of a work group or team. Traditionally, training in social work has been provided for individuals through courses leading to professional qualification. Post-qualifying and specialist training has also, typically, been provided on courses away from the workplace. But there is a growing realisation that providing the means for individuals to attain qualification—the traditional model for entry into most professions—may not be a sufficient training for residential and other forms of group-based care.

We write at a time of considerable debate and contention about the direction that training for residential care workers should take in the future. The issues concern how far current, generic social work courses leading to professional qualification provide a sufficient training for residential care that adequately covers the specialised needs of the different care groups, especially children and young people.

Training Cultures

The personal social services, in independent and public sectors, have had little tradition of developing services through job enhancement or investment in staff development. Social service departments, under the pressure of major policy developments, have more recently developed in-house training and used external courses but these moves, in most cases, fall short of any systematic approach to the development of staff. Unlike other service industries, personal and social care service agencies have tended to rest their faith in traditional courses rather than develop comprehensive, agency policies for training and the development of their workforce. This has led to the situation where few agencies have an approach to staff recruitment, training and development which integrates these functions with existing and changing operational and practice requirements of the service.

In relation to staffing, care agencies have tended to assume either that the competent worker can be recruited from qualifying courses—as is usually the case in field social work—or that the tasks associated with caring for people can be performed by suitably mature people (typically women) in the case of the basic-level residential care worker. These notions have, in turn, had an impact on the assumptions that care providers hold about the need for training and about who should provide this. To the extent that agencies have established training policies or priorities, these have concerned ensuring that particular specialisms are covered and that basic orientation courses are made available to new entrants. In terms of a training culture this can only be described as a piecemeal and somewhat marginal response to immediate organisational needs.

The general trend in social service department training units has been to allocate time and resources to providing in-house courses for specific staff (e.g. in response to new legislation). Seconding people on external courses is relatively expensive and has been seen as something for the benefit of the individual rather than a means of accessing knowledge and experience for wider dissemination within the agency.

There has been a considerable growth in the production and publication of training packages for use by individuals, groups and agencies. These cater for specialised requirements and offer cheap ways of meeting new demands. They are based in a belief in the cost effectiveness of pre-packaged kits. But off-the-shelf materials of this sort must raise questions about their relevance or about their adaptability by people who have little or no training expertise. To what extent do these materials help their users to locate the training within the wider contexts of, for example, changing demands on the home?—new agency policies or priorities?—the need for consistent practice within a staff group?—internal quality assurance procedures? or even to be clear about the purposes and value bases of the home? The NISW Programme developed a critical stance in relation to products of this sort (see Payne 1991a) and a framework to help people evaluate training materials (Phillipson, 1990).

Training and Quality of Service

In general we must note some ambivalence across the sectors but particularly in private homes, about the benefits of training. Although few would argue with the value of well trained staff and the important contribution that they make to the quality of the service, it is widely reported that, once qualified, staff tend to leave residential work in favour of field social work (Howe, 1992). This is clearly a disincentive since staff turnover is not only disruptive in terms of loss of continuity but costly in terms of loss of investment.

A general assumption that qualification and training ensures quality of service applies across the medical and caring professions. This assumption is being increasingly challenged, however, as users and consumers articulate alternative values, standards and requirements. Recent examples of malpractice suggest that professional peer review has a questionable record in ensuring quality. These trends lead to a general questioning of the nature and purposes of training and this applies as much to the provision of residential care as any other service. The NISW Programme entered into the research, as did all the CHI Programmes, with a clear mandate to take account of the needs and views of residents and their carers as well as to learn from the experience of grassroots and—given the profile of deployment of qualified staff in residential care—less trained practitioners. For these reasons there was always the possibility that the work of the Programme would challenge existing ways of looking at training.

The Challenge for the Programme

These were some of the issues which confronted the Programme and which affected the way the work could be developed. One of the key challenges was that training and staff development—as distinct from providing supervision for care workers—have not always been seen as a management responsibility. The development of NVQ has pushed managers and senior staff to think more clearly about training but, as noted earlier, primarily in relation to the individual learner.

In contrast, this Programme was based on the belief that practice development is an inherent part of service provision and, as such, a management responsibility. Individual and staff team support, ensuring the availability of appropriate training and development is thus an intrinsic aspect of management and part of an integrated approach to ensuring relevant, effective and good quality services.

The Programme implicitly explored the relevance of training which is geared to the individual carer and professional development on the one hand and that which emphasises team approaches and service-led development on the other.

Developing Training for Care Staff

The Aims of the Programme

The NISW researchers approached the work by defining a rather wider set of aims than those outlined in the DOH brief. As well as taking the basic-level care worker as the focus of training, the team looked at ways of defining team and individual training needs in relation to the purposes of the home as whole. The work specifically addressed the Wagner recommendation, therefore, that each home should have a coherent plan for the training of its staff.

The brief given to all Programmes was to develop models for general application. NISW followed an incremental, organic approach to the task rather than developing and testing one generic package. The product, in their terms, was a series of projects which modelled different possibilities in different agencies and contexts. Each was intended to stimulate wider local interest and extend locally, where possible, as well as to provide written materials for general dissemination. The production of a generic manual or package was not pursued until all projects were more or less completed in order that the project experience and the incremental learning could be incorporated.

The Value Base

The values underpinning the work of the NISW Programme were drawn not only from the principles and recommendations of the Wagner review but also from the previous work of NISW in developing training for a range of social work and care staff. The research was also firmly based in approaches to adult learning, education and training and in an understanding of the organisational contexts within which training and staff development are offered. The researchers took the view that training initiatives for basic-level care workers could not be thought about or put into practice in isolation from wider aspects of care provision and management (Douglas & Payne 1988).

The design and scope of the work were shaped by the following principles:

• training opportunities should be based in, and consistent with, the values, practice principles and purposes of the home and these should be made explicit;

• the resident has a central role in formulating the purposes and reviewing standards of the service and hence has a contribution to make in identifying training needs;

• staff training and development should be an integral part of service provision and quality assurance: training for care workers should be understood and planned within the broader frameworks of service development;

• managers should see the provision of training as part of their overall management responsibility;

• education and training should be integrated with practice: programmes should be designed or adapted for each establishment in order to ensure that training complements everyday practice. It follows that training needs should be defined with the involvement of the staff themselves;

• the continuity and coherence of residential care are based on staff who are able to work together as a team. Training should enhance team working;

• the climate for learning is of central importance and this should value existing skills and knowledge, shared learning and exchange of experience.

It follows, then, that the work was concerned as much with understanding the *contexts* within which learning and developmental opportunities are provided—the organisational climate, training policies and culture, management attitudes—and the *processes* of planning and providing training—as with the knowledge and skill content and the way these are packaged. The results of the work were thus intended to address how to create an appropriate climate and milieu for learning as well as provide guidelines on how to identify training needs, plan, design and run a training programme.

How the Work was Developed

The main source of ideas and practical experience came from a series of projects, each involving a number of care establishments, specifically designed and set up to explore different aspects of the task.

In all twenty-three projects, involving detailed work in collaboration with over 100 participant homes and agencies, were conducted which covered a range of care establishments and provided the Programme with wide frames of reference across care groups, sectors of provision, types of establishment, forms of intervention, levels of organisational support and range of objective (see Appendix 4.4).

Homes and agencies involved initially were recruited through an invitation in the trade journals. This drew a healthy number of enquiries from homes keen to explore ways of promoting training. These were not cynical responses. Our interviews with owners and managers suggested that the NISW projects provided people with the opportunity to pursue aspects of good practice which they had lacked the time or other resources to initiate by themselves.

Some additional projects were set up to cover specific areas of work. For example, the Programme wanted to ensure that topical issues were addressed in relation to homes for children and young people; that NVQ developments were taken into account; that some attention was given to the needs of black and ethnic minority groups and that mental health work was included.

In this way the work covered a range of interests but, as with other Programmes, the majority of projects were based in provision for elders.

The projects were interventionist, in that they aimed to produce change, but participative in that they worked from locally defined needs with care managers and workers rather than imposing change on them. But, as we have already noted, the Programme was promoting certain values which represented a critique of current approaches to training as well as seeking to incorporate good practice and principles for residential care.

The consultants who led the projects met regularly as a means of ensuring that there was an exchange of experience and information across the projects. It was evident from the discussions that took place at these meetings that there was a high level of consensus about best practice in providing training for care workers.

The aims of the projects were complex in that they were pursuing local aims as well as the general objectives of the Programme. In commenting on the work we have had to keep in mind the distinction between the developmental aims of the Programme—leading to the formulation of training approaches and other products for dissemination—and specific local aims which varied home by home, project by project.

The projects were grouped into clusters:

- those working with individual establishments

- those setting up or working with networks or consortia

- those working with an agency or local authority SSDs

- those concerned with evaluating training materials or courses.

Between them the projects covered a wide range of aspects and these included:

- how to evaluate training materials

- staff training in the private sector

- induction and foundation training in the private sector

- the role of training in quality assurance

- the role of managers as trainers

- work-based assessment for NVQ

- roles of SSD trainers in the independent sector

- staff training and the needs of African-Caribbean and Asian elders.

An account of the projects, their aims and scope is available in the Interim Report produced by the Programme (NISW 1991).

A Generalised Account of the Projects

The Programme adopted an approach to designing and running training programmes which built on a grassroots assessment of training needs.

Projects were led by independent consultants working within an agreed set of values. They were expected to contribute to the overall work of the Programme as well as to pursue locally determined aims.

There was no attempt to design and try out a single training package or programme: projects were expected to develop approaches that were appropriate to meet local needs and objectives. The aim was for partici- pant care homes or agencies to build from and adapt the NISW-led projects both 'in-house' and by creating links and networks with other care providers. Many of the projects were also set up to explore how the formation of networks for sharing resources and the exchange of training practice might be encouraged.

Although the projects were diverse they shared basic values and each followed a broadly similar pattern of activities. What follows is a gener- alised account of the way that the projects were set up and run.

Setting objectives
Each project set out with clear objectives which were negotiated with each participant home or agency. In all cases this involved discussion with the home managers and usually staff were also involved. In only a few cases were residents included at this point.

Auditing
Most projects were based on an appraisal of the current work of the home based on a questionnaire developed by the NISW Programme. This provided a way of identifying gaps or areas of practice that needed to change. The audit covered a number of areas:

The Purposes and Philosophy of the Home: One of the features of the audit was an emphasis on clarifying the aims, purposes and philosophy of the home. There were several examples where managers and staff discovered that they did not have a shared or detailed understanding of what the establishment was setting out to achieve.

Characteristics of the Home, the Residents and the Staff: The audit gathered basic information about the home, about the residents and staff. As well as physical details, the audit recorded indicators of the 'health' of the home in terms of, for example, staff turnover, levels of stress, communication difficulties, levels of and type of staff support.

Assessment of Quality and Current Care Practice: The audit tool asked various questions about care standards and practice and how these are reviewed. Many projects used a simple self-evaluation checklist (Payne and McLachlin 1989) as a means of inviting staff and residents to think about and discuss the running of the home. This was the point at which several homes included residents in the process.

An agenda for training
This appraisal was used to develop a profile of the kind of training needed to address the needs of the home as a whole and to decide on priorities.

Designing and running a training programme
Designing a programme for training involved thinking about the overall shape, size and duration of the training events, the content, the style and level of teaching/learning, about whether or not to use existing materials or packages, who should be involved and how the programme would be reviewed. This included decisions about leadership and the resources needed in terms of materials, staff time and cover, management involvement. The relative benefits of internal or external trainers was a point of discussion for most projects.

Outputs
Most of the projects provided an account of the work in the form of a review and most also published materials for wider circulation. These

represent a significant result of the collaboration of researchers and care home staff. Several projects also led to the involvement of more homes or agencies in the area and to plans for future work.

Models of Implementation

The work explored a number of different models of implementation which included multi-agency, cross sector and care group mixes and these provided valuable opportunities to explore collaboration across traditional boundaries. The work was developed in a variety of ways although each project adopted the basic approach outlined above.

Individual care homes

Managers and proprietors with specific objectives used the NISW Programme to plan and initiate staff training. These were establishments which had already decided on the value of training for care workers and anticipated immediate benefits (Wiseman 1991).

Clusters of care homes

Several projects involved groups of homes for one care group or from one department or agency. These included a group led by a senior officer with strategic objectives eg. for job enhancement; and promoting a quality initiative; a group wanting to develop training and recognition for care workers; building a reputation for quality through training; and developing 'in-house' training materials.

An example of this model is that of an independent agency recently hived off from the local authority. Training consultants were given a contract to plan and carry out a comprehensive training programme for the staff of a group of homes for elders. The agency policy was to 'go for quality' as a means of establishing its reputation and securing future contracts with the local authority. The physical condition and environment of the homes were highly important but staff development was seen as the only means of improving the practice and the quality of care. As a result, a considerable amount of time and money was invested in training. The NISW project supported work in three homes where a programme of training involving senior and care staff was worked out. Each was somewhat different but in all cases the aim was to promote a strong awareness of the needs and rights of the residents and to break away from some of the more traditional and restrictive regimes that had typified a few of the homes. The training events were in-house, mostly led by senior staff with support from the consultants and were fully participative. They were based on *Homes Are For Living In* (DOH/SSI, 1989a) which was used as a broad frame for thinking about current practice.

The agency commitment meant that, although this was a participative approach, the work was understood and supported throughout the organisation. Homes could learn from each other and staff had a stronger identity as care workers within the agency. As a management strategy there were obvious advantages for a new organisation in developing a corporate ethos through a coherent training approach (Daley et al 1992, Kelcey 1992).

Mixed private care home consortia
Here groups of owner-proprietors used the Programme to explore their training needs, pool resources and produce relevant training materials. (Mabon 1991a and b).

An example of this model was a group of twelve private homes from a care home association which got together to pool ideas and resources for providing basic training for their care staff. One of the proprietors acted as consultant and convenor for the group. This project proceeded more slowly than some. The different needs and resources of the homes meant that it took a while for people to clarify what was wanted and how to pursue it but it was clear that homes benefited from the exchange of ideas.

Inter-agency networks of residential facilities for a particular care group
Here several agencies worked together with the aim of sharing resources and enhancing communication between them. An example of this model was the link between a social services training department and a group of voluntary agencies in the field of mental health. The local authority ran no services for people with mental health problems and offered to support the voluntary agencies through a training programme. The Programme was used as a way of getting started—to plan and pilot an introductory programme for basic-level mental health workers.

The agencies were already members of a strong network of services in the area and it was relatively easy for the managers to come together and plan a strategy.

The model was worked out in a steering group consisting of the SSD trainer, the NISW consultant and representatives of most of the agencies. The aim was to provide a foundation course which each agency could nominate staff to attend. Each course member would be supported by a mentor from their home or agency and each would be expected to involve their colleagues in discussions or exercises arising from the sessions. In this way it was intended that the course would act as a stimulus for wider staff development and agency learning. The course was designed to be interactive, to help people learn from their own experience and from each other rather than provide formal teaching. The agency managers agreed that information about mental illness was not what was needed: the staff would benefit more from discussing their feelings and experience (Peretz and Payne forthcoming).

The course was successful in helping people to look at their under-standing of mental illness, to challenge some aspects of practice, to build a sense of identity and expertise and to take more account of the needs of residents. It was also appreciated because it gave people an opportunity to find out about the work of others and explore other perspectives on mental health. It was less successful in reaching and influencing the wider staff groups but there was enthusiasm for running the programme again. The existing links between agency managers meant that there was a level of trust and an open exchange in evaluating the results of the training.

Individual homes linked through a consultant
Here contact between individual homes was minimal or non-existent but they were aware that other establishments were working with the same consultant.

One project, for example, aimed to provide in-house training and support for staff in homes for children and young people in one local authority and involved a consultant and an SSD training officer. The homes worked separately but some of their common concerns became apparent to the external consultant and the trainer.

College staff as consultants for home-based training
Here college teaching staff from social work and related courses were used as consultants and the potential role of college staff in providing in-house, tailor-made training was looked at.

An example here was the consultancy offered by a college to a small group of private care homes. Originally it was planned that the group might share resources but the differences between them made this impracticable. A key difference was the extent to which the homes had any awareness of training developments and this was linked with their level of involvement with local or national training networks. This project was interesting in that one of the unintended spin-offs was that the consultant became the source of information exchange between the homes and built up her expertise as a college-based trainer.

In another project a college lecturer was involved in running some of the in-house sessions. The experience led to a discussion about the difference between home- and college-based learning opportunities and the difference between individual and team-based teaching (Miller T. 1991).

These, then, were some of the ways that the projects were organised. They allowed the Programme to explore some of the issues involved in making links across sectors, institutions and care groups as well as gaining perspectives on a variety of ways in which training can be planned and supported.

Training Approaches
The projects also used a range of training options and styles, including in-house, self designed approaches and external training opportunities.

Several projects developed *in-house training*, through planning and designing their own activities with consultant support, or by using and adapting published materials. The focus tended to be on supporting the home manager in developing and co-ordinating an appropriate in-house programme: the NISW consultants were not primarily there to provide training. A number of establishments were keen to establish NVQ for their workers and some projects involved preparation for this.

The *external approaches* used involved short courses or training days provided by the agency or local college which were geared towards team-based learning. In some projects, care workers from different establishments shared these opportunities. Because the intention was to emphasise team-based development, the Programme did not include college-based or professional courses but did include trials of some open learning packages. A major advantage of external options were the chances provided for workers to consider other views and to have their own attitudes challenged. An in-house programme without an external mentor of some sort could, for example, fail to question existing practices or to boost staff confidence and motivation.

A smaller number of staff, in private homes for elders and in children's homes, used *open learning courses*. Packages were provided and learning support provided by workplace mentors, with guidance from project consultants. These demonstrated how support in the home from more experienced staff and from fellow students significantly increased both the personal and practice impact of these courses. Where the course was well integrated with in-house training and activity, it was far more likely to be completed by the candidate and to have a positive impact in the establishment.

Several establishments were interested in pursuing NVQ as a means of demonstrating quality. The NISW projects provided an opportunity for managers and senior workers to explore the competencies and training required to support NVQ accreditation. Independent homes, which tended to lack a tradition of training, were helped to assess existing competencies and focus on the role that more experienced staff could play in providing for less experienced colleagues. This was useful in building up confidence, in making knowledge and assumptions more explicit and giving formal acknowledgement for practice-based learning. Where several workers were assessed together, it gave the opportunity for discussion and reflection. Unlike the other projects, however, there was a tendency for the NVQ-based work to confirm rather than challenge traditional practices.

The Experience of the Projects

We look now at the experience of the projects and at some of the issues that arose from them. Here we are mainly concerned with the practicalities and processes involved: we consider the results of the project, how far they achieved their objectives and the benefit for residents in the next section.

How did the participant homes and agencies get on? What were the significant issues about using the NISW approach? What helps or hinders the process? What about the costs and resources involved?

Attitudes to Training

Attitudes to staff training were complex and sometimes there were conflicting views within one home. For example, staff training was pursued:

- to develop good quality care;

- to demonstrate that the home was concerned to ensure quality services;

- because training was seen as a quality indicator;

- for care workers to achieve certification (eg NVQ);

- to motivate staff and improve morale;

- to reduce staff turnover and retain good staff through the 'reward' of training.

But at the same time there were managers who:

- wanted to minimise costs of training;

- held the view that caring, experience and maturity are better than training;

- thought training could interfere with natural caring abilities;

- feared formal educational methods;

- held doubts about the relevance of training for the real work of their home;

- were concerned that trained staff would move on or demand higher wages.

Interviews with care workers in several homes showed that the advent of a training initiative was, not surprisingly, viewed with some suspicion: were they being 'fattened up' for sale? Were they being told they were incompetent? Would they be expected to take more responsibility?

Care staff held a range of ideas about training: a significant number expressed doubts about its usefulness or their own ability to benefit. Others viewed it as an opportunity to develop their work positively. It was common for people to see training in a very formal sense, associated with educational institutions rather than caring work. Before starting the training, most staff expressed some doubts which varied quite widely depending on their own previous experience and their perceptions of the role and responsibilities of people who they saw as 'qualified' or 'trained'. Scepticism and fears included the following views and questions:

- is it worth the time?

- will it be too intellectual to cope with?

- is it necessary?—the work is really a question of relating to people as fellow human beings

- you can be too trained

- if we're doing a good job, why do we need training?

- training might mean I have to take more responsibility

- I don't want to have to make decisions about difficult people.

There were positive responses too:

- you do need special knowledge and information for your work

- its good to meet others in the field

- it is an opportunity to reflect

- I want specific information and ideas about how to approach people

- I like the idea of learning about what other people do

- It means we do have special skills and some status.

Support for the Work

All the projects were supported, if not actively led, by consultants appointed by the Programme. In all cases the decision to participate involved the home proprietor or manager and, in most cases had either been initiated or agreed by senior managers. Where projects involved collaboration between homes or between agencies a process of negotiation—not always led by the consultant—ensured that in most cases there was a clarity about the aims and implications of joint work. Agreement for the work from senior staff or the wider agency was not problematic on the whole.

It was not always the case, however, that there was active support for the projects at senior level. There were a few examples where senior staff had not foreseen the impact that a grassroots approach might have on the agency as a whole. Equally, where a training unit of a SSD had negotiated a project with care homes, operational managers were not always fully aware of the possible implications for their work.

Within the homes, frontline and junior staff were not always involved in the decision to pursue a training initiative. Some staff, for example, found themselves expected to attend courses designed by others as part of a wider exercise in collaboration and resource sharing with other agencies. Such incidents ran counter to the overall philosophy of assessing training needs in discussion with staff to ensure their commitment through a sense of ownership.

Assessing Current Practice and the Training Needs of the Home

In general, the idea of starting with a look at the current work and practice of the home was appreciated and welcomed. It helped managers and staff to stand back and consider their work and it was an opportunity to involve a range of people in review. It appeared broadly successful in encouraging people to look at the home as a whole.

A fundamental problem was in ensuring that the audit process was used in a way that distinguished between issues for management and issues for training. This depended on who was steering the audit process and who was involved in interpreting the results. The project experience pointed to the benefit of training plans being considered alongside general plans for development and, therefore, the need to involve management at an appropriate level.

Like most tools of this sort, the audit was dependent on the commitment and confidence of those using it. Many people found the audit document produced by the Programme too lengthy and detailed. The purpose of using it was not always clear and there were some who thought it was for the research rather than for the benefit of the home. Private homes in one project, for example, took between five weeks to a year to complete the process and there was doubt about its usefulness. One difficulty was that some home managers were not able to recognise the implications of the information collected for training and staff development.

The process involved interpretation, selection and prioritising: which training needs expressed by staff should be pursued? How were staff views to be understood in terms of the needs of the home as a whole? There were, for example, at least two home managers who were dismayed at yet more staff requests for training on lifting when they would rather staff were better equipped to meet the residents' needs for bereavement counselling. What did the request for lifting mean?

The use of specific tools to aid discussion and reflection on practice was generally welcomed by home staff where they were used. The self-evaluation checklist (Payne and McLachlin, 1989), guides managers, staff and residents in looking at different aspects of life in the home using a simple point scoring system. People found this easy to use and interpret and were prepared to reflect on the inconsistencies, differences in perception and priorities that the exercise revealed between different groups of people. The value of the checklist, however, depended on the extent to which the results were used as the basis for discussion at all levels within the home—including residents, night staff, domestics, care officers and managers—and then translated into plans and action. The checklist assumes the interests of the resident to be central and this was generally welcomed and accepted. It helped to promote user values as the frame of reference for making decisions and selecting between conflicting ideas.

Some project consultants used other techniques—for example an exercise which uses 'a day in the life' of a lounge to record the nature and levels of activity and interaction was used as a basis of discussion, planning and review.

Planning and Running the Programme

Most of the projects designed a training plan and programme tailor made for the individual home or cluster of homes.

The decisions involved in planning and designing a programme related to: the aims of training; the level and main focus of the content; the materials to be used; the timing and duration of the programme; who should attend; teaching and learning methods; who should teach/lead; the pros and cons of internal events or external courses; the resource implications. In many respects answering such questions required an experienced trainer. The consultants certainly took a lead—in collaboration with agency trainers where they were also involved—in helping to decide such issues. The project experience raised important questions about how far a set of guidelines or principles for practice, or a manual, can steer managers or others though this process. It was clear that assessing training needs and producing a plan for action required considerable discussion, thought and a degree of specialised knowledge about methods, approaches and processes of training.

The work undertaken on how to evaluate training materials was, perhaps, underexploited by the projects (Phillipson, 1990). Advice and guidance on assessing the relevance, authority and usefulness of different publications could be of considerable value to individual managers.

What Helps or Hinders Application of Course Learning?
Commentary from managers and staff suggests that there were several aspects of the projects which helped to ensure that the training was relevant and a legitimate use of time and resources:

- staff needed confidence in the training: having a hand in its design and content clearly helped;

- individuals needed to understand the nature of the training they are being asked to follow: lack of clarity about its form or purpose acted against their openness to learning;

- colleagues needed to understand their place in the overall scheme of a training programme—both in terms of specific aspects and in relation to general staff development;

- being able to take on new perspectives depended quite heavily on the relationship between colleagues—some feelings and views (envy, resentment, misunderstanding) can be a real bar;

- any mismatch between wider agency values and traditions and the ethos of a course can result in tensions: exposing people to new ways of thinking and learning can lead to difficulties for the individual staff member;

- a network approach can provide a forum in which agencies and individuals can have confidence.

Resident Involvement
How far were the projects able to involve residents in looking at the running of the home and setting the agenda for training? Placing residents' interests first was almost universally accepted in principle but, in practice, residents' involvement tended to be limited. Their interests were considered but according to staff perceptions of their needs and views rather than by direct consultation.

Overall, few projects involved residents directly—either in guiding objectives or commenting on the impact of training work—this is something that project workers could have explored more systematically.

However, residents were actively involved in some projects and these provided practical examples that could be considered for wider application:

- residents were interviewed about their life in the home at the same time that training plans were being discussed. However, this usually fell short of seeking their direct comment or involvement in guiding training objectives;

- residents carried out the self-evaluation checklist exercise and comparison of their views with those of staff proved useful;

- people with learning disabilities were involved in training with the staff—an approach which was also tried successfully in an SCA project;

- elders in one home were invited to participate in a video role play exercise with staff;

- in some homes, residents were asked to comment after the training: they were able to give their views of whether the work had made a positive impact in the home.

Residents were also involved in less direct ways: project consultants, for example, worked shifts and made visits to meet people and get a feel of the place; informal discussions with residents proved to be useful for consultants to understand something about what matters to residents in the home.

Relevance to Different Care Groups
Project experience suggested that it is possible and desirable to develop an approach which is generic but which allows more specialised materials to be included within the training programme.

What happened in most cases was that an overall approach and structure was decided upon together with the key areas which the learning events would cover. The generic—or *core aspects* were, as we have seen, the involvement of staff and a basic audit process which aimed to generate a training agenda that would help to pursue the purposes and goals of the home as a whole. *Specific aspects* were then addressed by developing materials or using existing packages.

Generic approaches can lead to creative reconsideration of models for one care group in the light of other traditions. For example, normalisation principles have been developed furthest in services for people with learning disabilities although they were intended to be used in all services where segregation, isolation or stigma might be an issue. Similarly ideas about promoting personal development and independence, well established in ideals for child care, could be refreshing in the field of care for elders.

However, we noted a danger in assuming that any published or pre-packaged materials are generic. Experience in the projects confirmed that many packs intended as generic, were rooted in ideas of care for elders. The case of NVQ is instructive. Although styled as generic, the competencies originally developed by the Care Sector Consortium had a strong focus on care for elders. Workers in establishments for young adults found that the materials used in NVQ tended to assume dependency and that workers would have a physical care-taking role: they needed to adapt a large proportion of the competency framework to their context and styles of work and felt unsure how, or how far, they could do this. Similarly, workers in homes for people with learning difficulties, using a (generic) open learning package, felt it was really designed with care for elders in mind. They found it unchallenging in some ways and unable fully to reflect the scope of their work.

There is, then, a case for developing special training inputs and a number of projects published their own materials for this reason.

Given these differences in philosophies of work, as well as differing resident needs and interests, it was important that projects covered a range of establishment types/care groups and this was reflected in the Programme's publications. The development around training for work with people with dementia is important since staff working in most establishments for older people need to understand and deal with this problem. Experience with a specialist home for people with Alzheimer's Syndrome suggested that staff have few training resources and little encouragement to work in line with the resident-centred principles of this Programme. While residents were well cared for and staff conscientious, little was offered to enhance or maintain the residents' capacity to make choices.

The gap in the Programme was in relation to care for people with drug or alcohol problems. There were, as a result, few homes offering a therapeutic environment. Those that were involved were interesting in that they rely on team-based approaches in which there is a clear set of working principles with training back up but they, too, valued the opportunity, entailed in the NISW projects, to review working methods and philosophies.

There were also relatively few homes catering for younger adults with physical disabilities, where staff may be working in a very different way to those in homes for older people.

The Programme was able to include projects catering specifically for black elders which included all sectors. This was crucial in understanding some of the issues for black residents and staff and those from other ethnic minorities. Although they are not a separate group in any way, their needs have been so poorly catered for in mainstream homes, particularly those for elders, that a need for specialist homes has been recognised.

Relevance to Sectors of Provision

The projects covered the three sectors of provision and a range of establishment types within them. Generally, there were few distinctions across the sectors in relation to training and staff development needs. Differences related rather more to whether a home was an individual establishment or part of a wider organisation and whether or not they were connected to local or national training networks. The issues concerned who was able to set the agenda, design and resource a programme to meet training needs. Individual private homes, for example, were more likely to be isolated from wider supports or influences. Although more critical about the need for training, many recognised the value of the in-house and grounded nature of the projects. Owners and proprietors could ensure they retained control of the agenda for training and its costs.

We noted earlier that as well as developing training networks the Programme made some progress in demonstrating the scope for co-operation between sectors. In the independent sector there has been development of training networks in themselves, and encouragement of the role of local care associations in supporting training and other quality assurance developments. A few projects took the Local Authority area as a base and drew interested participants from all sectors: one aimed to contribute to an area-wide strategy for services for people with learning disabilities.

Can the Approach Stand Alone?

The project experience suggested that the main issue in relation to the implementation of the NISW approach was the availability of particular knowledge and skills.

The critical task was that of linking training needs with the needs of the service—the home as a whole. The first element in this was to undertake a review of the home and consider the training implications that this reveals. The main difficulties here arose in translating the need for operational or practice changes into training requirements. To be useful for care managers a manual would have to help them with this process. Our follow-up visits and interviews suggested that the individual care home could undertake this assessment element: the link to quality review was strong and the potential benefit of doing this was clear. Translating the outcomes of this kind of exercise into an agenda for training looked more difficult. Doing so within a framework of values that promotes resident and staff rights to participation added to the complexity. There are two main issues.

First, given dominant attitudes to training, staff are likely to see training as providing them with concrete skills and knowledge to meet their immediate needs in terms of health and safety at work and the more physical aspects of the care task. The request for lifting skills was a helpful reminder that staff are right to think about their own interests. What help does a manager require to balance the interests of individual staff and a staff team? and the interests of residents and staff?

Tensions were sometimes evident between the view taken by management and the views expressed by staff, between agency policies for training and grassroots definitions of training needs. Ideas about care, choice or resident-centred practice can vary: consultants had to make their own values explicit and to negotiate these ideas with participants, in line with principles of adult learning—the need for people to 'own' their learning for it to be sustained and put into practice. How might home proprietors and managers fare without someone from 'outside' to help?

The second set of issues related to the knowledge, skills and practical experience needed to plan and design an appropriate training programme. Can a manual take the place of the consultants who, on the whole, provided this support for the projects? The role of the consultant here was a crucial one. All the projects relied on some help from outside to develop suitable programmes. Staff and managers were usually clear about the focus of training they wanted and how this would enhance the service: few were confident about how best to proceed from there. This points to in-house initiatives needing at least some specialised help in designing and running training events.

Our discussions with consultants showed that their essential contribution was in the area of designing adult educational opportunities. This was not so much about the *content* of training but about the *manner and milieu* in which learning is provided. How often and where should sessions take place? How much and what sort of content is appropriate? How to conduct training sessions? How many people to have in a group? What kind of things can people best learn from each other and when to use an outside expert? Helping people to think through these questions addressed issues for everyday staff management and relationships.

The experience of the collective projects—consortia, networks and clusters of homes from one agency—showed the value of peer support. Information exchange and help with problem solving was as important as the sharing of resources. Each did require a form of leadership but this was as much about convening meetings and attending to basic communication as with providing a vision or clear direction for the work. The sense of isolation among small homes—in independent and public sectors—that we noted across CHI points to the benefit of homes coming together to pursue common training and perhaps other needs.

Resources and Materials

The resources needed by the projects were mostly associated with staff and trainer time, the opportunity to discuss plans with the right combination of people and cover for people attending training events. Materials used in the projects were either:

- published training materials suitably adapted;

- frameworks such as NVQ or established open learning courses;

- materials developed by project workers.

Many projects made use of existing training materials and packages but the programmes did not rely on these. Effective learning was more than a matter of transferring knowledge and much attention was given to the kind of setting and the supports needed to create an appropriate learning environment.

Resources of time, knowledge and support were needed for implementation. Managers needed not only budgets but access to advice and ideas from their peers, line managers or other professionals. The use of networks, therefore, was important in encouraging establishments to get started and to sustain the work in the longer term. Equally, establishments which lacked basic stability in management and organisational structure were unlikely to be able to pursue effective training.

The Programme published guidance on how to select and use off-the-shelf materials (Phillipson 1990, Hillyard-Parker et al 1993). The need for this information was confirmed in our discussions with managers and care staff, who often know little about what is available and who have limited funds with which to try different options.

Many of the projects produced their own materials. These may have a particular appeal for private sector homes since many were developed in collaboration with small home owners.

Value for Money

An overall view of value for money was assessed by looking at the different models tried across the Programme as a whole and with other available models—such as external training courses.

Value for money was considered in relation to the benefits of each project and the costs in terms of time, effort and money.

The main requirements for the training projects were:

• staff time in planning and attending training events: this varied but was significant where team-based approaches were used. The time implications were reduced where training events doubled with or were complemented by using staff meetings;

• staff cover: again cover for people in training was a significant resource issue and did require extra funds in some cases;

• managers' time in planning and running the project;

• time and cost of support and advice: in many cases an external person was appointed to support the work. The time and money costs of this varied but usually this role was taken on by an internal trainer or senior manager. These people were available both from within the agency and from other agencies. The resource implications were usually those of time rather than direct money cost;

• cost of course materials and equipment: costs for training materials were generally low.

All staff time has to be paid for, but how far the input was perceived as a cost depended on the situation. In some settings training was viewed as an intrinsic part of running the service; in others, it was seen as an extra cost—a common view in private sector homes. Some local authority homes held a training budget but still saw the cost as something separate from the ordinary running of the home.

Management approaches and attitudes had an impact on the actual and felt costs of training. Where training was integrated with practice it was not seen as costly, partly because it was easier to make time available for training events and partly because the dividing line between 'training' and reflecting on the work in day-by-day discussion, staff meetings and supervision was harder to define.

The range of projects allowed useful comparison of the different options on a value-for-money basis. While in-house approaches were particularly cost effective, managers still needed to allow for staff cover. Projects which used some form of external support and integrated this with in-house and practice-based learning, were likely to have a greater impact. In-house sessions were useful for team development, for confidence and application to practice whereas external sessions or courses (including open learning) were useful for introducing fresh perspectives, challenging assumptions and making contact with others.

Team-based approaches, whether in-house or externally run were useful for practice. On the whole, in-house training was considered to be the most cost effective: generally, work could be done at the cost of providing staff cover for training sessions and for a facilitator where the training was not organised by someone from within the agency. Normal supervision, handover sessions, paired working and guidance on the job were also used to back up the formal training.

The Outcomes of the Projects

Here we consider what happened in the projects. Did they succeed in their own terms? Did they help to meet local objectives? What were the outcomes for staff and for residents? Did the projects demonstrate that attention to staff training helps to improve care practice and to ensure quality of life for residents?

Outcomes for the Care Establishment

The NISW approach emphasised that training should be linked to the overall tasks and purposes of the home. One of the interesting issues to emerge from this was the number of projects where the purposes of the home were not clear or not understood in the same way by all staff. Differences were revealed in the way people thought about the care task, about the way they should be working, about the needs of the residents—all fundamental issues to resolve if people are to work together effectively. In one project the audit process showed how lack of understanding was contributing to the considerable difficulties of staff in homes for children and young people.

In a sense this was an unintended outcome of the process. But this basic sorting out of ideas showed that there needs to be a consistency between the general aims of the service and staff practice. The implications for practice and training were obvious. For example, where the purpose of a small home was to help older mentally ill people to live as independently as possible it was confusing and frustrating that it was administrative staff who held information about residents' pensions and savings.

The clarification of purposes also brought new ideas and perspectives—many of which resulted from a more resident-focused orientation. The more staff were encouraged to think about what life in the establishment might be like for the resident, the more ideas about the care task tended to shift. Although there were many staff who wanted help with the more concrete and physical side of the care task, it was also clear that staff valued help with understanding the experience of people with mental health problems, dealing with death and bereavement, or stress management. These kind of topics signalled, perhaps, an awareness and willingness to deal not only with staff needs in coping with the emotional impact of the work but also recognising something about the experience and needs of residents. This opening up of the agenda for training seemed to us to be significant in reaching a more shared understanding with residents about what matters most to them.

A further unexpected outcome, in some cases, was a realisation that staff brought together for training purposes communicated rather more freely and creatively than they did in staff meetings or other occasions when their views and comments were sought by senior staff or external managers. Some homes were able to reflect, with the NISW consultant's help, on the kind of climate and support that encouraged staff to participate in this way.

One of the more general outcomes which we noted across all types of projects was the link between staff involvement in discussing and setting the training agenda, opportunities to discuss and reflect with colleagues in house and an increase in staff confidence and morale. Even where project work brought tensions out into the open, there was some relief that such difficulties were being recognised. It is not possible to comment with any authority on whether such changes will be sustained. Much might depend, for example, on how issues relating to training and opportunities for staff development were understood and taken up by managers after the project work ended. The indications were that the leadership role exercised by the head of home—whether or not part of a wider organisation—was crucial here.

Outcomes for Residents
There were two ways in which the training projects had an impact for residents. First there were projects where residents were involved in some way—either in an appraisal of the home or by commenting after the

training events. In these projects it was clear that residents gained direct benefits from a sense of participation and from knowing what was going on even if they did not influence the training agenda very markedly. This kind of outcome in a way reflected a management and staff outlook which already recognised not only the benefits to residents themselves of being more involved but also the advantages for the home as a whole.

The second way in which residents benefited was from changes in care practice, staff or management attitudes. The evidence here was rather harder to obtain since, in most cases, residents were unaware that any training was taking place or that anything different was happening. However, in most of the projects we visited, there were indications that staff had gained greater sensitivity and were more receptive to residents' needs and interests. It seemed that relationships between staff and residents had become more relaxed and certainly several residents implied that there had been some kind of 'sea change' in their carers' attitudes. Small changes can be indicative of more fundamental shifts. For example, in one home with a number of very frail and confused elders, each resident now has their own door key. Staff anxieties about lost keys and people being locked in or out were discussed in relation to residents' rights, staff responsibilities and risk taking: the issues involved were understood and accepted by all. The delight of one of the residents was expressed jokingly 'I'm twenty-one again!' In the same establishment a staff member thought that because she and her colleagues had a greater awareness and understanding of dementia this had led to rather less disturbed and wandering behaviour from one or two of the residents. It seemed that, when staff were less anxious, this communicated itself to the residents who, in turn, felt less anxious. There were examples, too, where staff had begun to do things *with* residents rather than *for* them: they had realised that there was more to tidying a resident's room than getting the job done. Such examples are small but important in demonstrating how a reappraisal of the care task through in-house discussion with fellow workers can result in significant outcomes for residents.

Outcomes for Care Staff

The Programme centred on staff training, as individuals and as a team. All the projects produced clear evidence of the kind of beneficial effects that training can have. These effects were, perhaps, most marked in raising morale and general confidence, helping people to be clearer about the kind of care that was appropriate for their particular residents, shifting attitudes and expectations, enabling people to move away from old regimes and to embrace new perspectives. The generally participative way that the training was set up increased the sense of responsibility for, and involvement in, providing a quality service.

We noted widespread caution among care workers about the reasons for training and about the likely benefits for them. In the event, however, most of those interviewed after a training project had responded well to the educational approaches taken in the training programmes. It did seem that staff reflecting together on their own and each other's work increased the level of sensitivity to residents and their needs. The staff appreciated the time to talk and became more supportive of each other. There appeared to be less anxiety about 'doing-it-the-way-it-has-always-been-done' and more freedom to ask and make arrangements with the residents themselves. One highly sceptical member of staff was surprised to find she appreciated the chance to listen to others: another was prompted to think it was time she wrote a book. Most care staff were enthusiastic about in-house training because it involved their colleagues. Comments by staff attending training sessions and at the end of programmes were generally positive. One of the recurrent themes was the enjoyment and learning that came from discussing practice with colleagues and peers.

There were several dimensions to this. One flowed from a sense of shared identity. In a mental health project, for example, where the workers came from different voluntary agencies one of the benefits referred to was that everyone was concerned with the same care group and a similar set of issues.

Another important benefit was that staff began to recognise and value their own experience. The notion that training always comes from outsiders gave way to an appreciation of the wisdom that people build up through practice. The rise in confidence and interest in the job that resulted from this kind of experience was clear in most of the projects—in this and in other Programmes where staff had the opportunity to talk about their work in an unthreatening way.

A third benefit was that staff made connections across boundaries: day and night staff met, staff from different homes met up, staff from different agencies learnt about one another's work.

Reflecting on and learning about things in-house enabled some staff to take on new perspectives but put some people under new pressures. There were certainly some staff who learnt to join in but who did not give up old attitudes: they retained a loyalty to a former regime while apparently accepting a new emphasis on, for example, resident choice. This kind of example alerts us to a need for some caution in relation to in-house team-based training: group pressure can lead people to appear to conform although they may have considerable doubts.

On the other hand, it was also clear that concentrated, in-house discussions and training events could expose individual and staff group difficulties. There is certainly a careful judgement to be made in some places as to whether training is an appropriate means of tackling particular difficulties.

The most important residual value for individuals and staff groups may well flow from sharing ideas and experience and having these validated.

The anxieties about change and caution about the meaning of training highlight the importance of involving staff in general management plans— not only those relating to training.

Local Outcomes

We noted that several projects were intended to develop wider links and extend the work to other homes or agencies. It was not only the consortia and clusters of homes which succeeded in bringing homes together to share ideas and training resources. Within SSDs for example, when other care home managers knew of the training initiative they were interested in joining in. In one case their work was extended to include day centres. Such developments highlight both the interest in training on the one hand and the willingness to link up across care homes—and in many cases— agency boundaries.

Programme Outputs

The work of the Programme is available in a number of publications since many projects produced reports, articles and training materials for wider circulation. These include induction and foundation training manuals, critical commentaries of the projects, descriptive accounts and evaluation materials. Many of these have been referenced in our account of the projects and developmental work.

At the general level the Programme produced a two-page evaluation chart in Care Weekly to enable individual homes to check their approaches and ideas about training. It helps managers and staff to identify areas for improvement or change and encourages the development of a training plan for the home (Payne 1992).

The main Programme publication is a comprehensive manual which guides care home managers and proprietors through the process of assessing their training needs and developing a training plan (Hillyard-Parker et al, 1993).

This draws on project experience up to the point of designing a programme of training. The manual provides a step-by-step guide through a sequence of tasks and activities:

- building a picture of the current work of the home

- assessing training needs from this

- deciding on priorities for training

- setting aims and objectives

- designing a programme

- evaluating the plan.

The approach is broadly the same as that followed in the projects, with detailed materials to help people through a complex set of tasks. In doing so it covers many of the points of difficulty identified from the projects. Each section includes an explanation of what needs to be done and why, a series of activities to be followed, practical ideas and examples.

One of the issues on which the manual provides clear guidance is that of working out the training implications that arise from an assessment of the home.

The guide includes many references to residents and the benefits of including them in the activities—as a way of understanding their needs and as a means of ensuring that residents views are heard and valued. The position of the residents is not, however, given prominence in the same way that, for example, the IQA review places residents' interests as central.

The work of the Programme also led to the setting up, in collaboration with SCA and others, of the Social Care Practice Centre. One of its main objectives is the exchange of information and training resources.

Discussion

In commenting on the work of the Programme we look at four main issues. First we discuss the contribution which the Programme makes to issues of providing and assuring quality services and, in particular, services which are relevant to and take account of user interests. Next we look at the work of this Programme in relation to other training approaches. Third, we consider some of the wider implications of the incremental approach which the Programme adopted and, in particular, how this has led to extensions of the work and collaboration between sectors. Finally, we consider the implications of the work for training and management.

Training and Quality

An underlying assumption of the work of this Programme was that investment in training would contribute to service quality and in two main ways: by ensuring that basic-level workers had relevant knowledge and skills for their work and by contributing more generally to staff morale by increasing workers' sense of their own value. We noted that the NISW approach placed emphasis upon the development of a training pro-gramme for an establishment which reflected the purposes and current needs of the home as a whole. Setting a training agenda was, therefore, concerned with the training needs of a work group as well as individual staff. The relationship between the definition of training needs and designing a programme to meet them on the one hand, and standards of service that meet residents' needs on the other was not, on the whole, explicitly explored through the projects. There was a general assumption that quality of service would follow from looking at the needs of the home as a whole. Generally the projects encouraged staff to take a more resident-focused look at their work and this did seem to result in new perspectives and new ideas about care tasks. The guidelines produced by NISW emphasised the importance of resident involvement and indicated some of the ways in which this might be made possible.

One of the most important contributions of this Programme should, perhaps, be seen in relation to the development of the workplace as a whole and the extent to which opportunities for staff team learning can lead to new perspectives and new practices. Investment in staff, in this context, had less to do with enhancing individual performance than with helping a work group to look more comprehensively at changing demands and expectations and how these can be met. This, in turn, creates an opening for the entry of user interests.

Training for Care Workers and Other Training Approaches

We discussed earlier how the approach pursued by the Programme stood in contrast to some traditional approaches and ideas about training on the one hand and new training developments, like NVQ, on the other. We suggested that the NISW approach was one which located training firmly in relation to service provision and development and at the level of the care home. As such this was a service-based approach rather than one which set out to meet individual training needs or more general strategic staff development interests. There are clear links between this work and the development of a competent work place as the basis for NVQ accreditation. A number of benefits have been demonstrated from this approach— the main one being the way in which training agendas can be set in relation to local needs, demands and objectives. The issue remains, however, as to how far the NISW approach is complementary to or stand in tension with other training opportunities and systems.

A Grassroots Approach and Collaboration Between Sectors

We mentioned earlier that many projects extended beyond the original participants to include other homes, agencies and sectors. This extension of the work partly followed existing contacts and relationships but there were also examples of managers wanting to join in something going on in this area.

The Programme has shown that a high level of collaboration within and between sectors is possible although the most successful examples were those that were able to build on existing networks. Good relationships were built up between agencies and across sectors but the extent to which people were then able to share or pool training resources was somewhat limited. The projects were often resourced by the NISW consultant and, to some extent, relied on their knowledge and initiative to draw suitable materials into the programme. Nevertheless, there was strong commitment to the idea of pooling resources and working together: the private care consortium and the mental health network, for example, are currently continuing the programmes they developed.

The benefits were clear from the level of staff interest in the work of other homes and other agencies. It seemed in all cases that the morale and interest of staff was greatly increased by these kinds of contact.

However, the work also revealed the lack of understanding and knowledge that can exist between SSDs and the independent sector— private homes in particular. The relationship between the independent sector and the SSD emerged as an important factor in the extent to which collaborative work could be pursued. One of the areas of difficulty was that proprietors were cautious that there might be links between a SSD training unit and the Inspection unit. They were concerned about confidentiality: would the trainers report to the inspectors?

We note here that the role of the consultant was often crucial in clarifying objectives and keeping contact straight. It appeared that trainers in social service departments were not used to taking a strong lead in helping managers to clarify their objectives or to make distinctions between management and training tasks.

Training and Management

One of the overall conclusions to be drawn from the experience of this Programme of development work has been well summed up by Chris Payne who headed the research:

> 'Our work suggests that the crucial factors determining effective application of learning lie much more within the workplace than the training situation.'

> (Payne, 1991b).

He makes three points which we would endorse.

First, that training should not be seen as something that can be 'bolted on' as an added activity that may be intended to bring about benefits—in changed care practices or staff attitudes, in the cohesion of a staff team— without taking account of the circumstances of the home and the context in which training is offered (Payne, 1991b).

Second, attitudes and the climate of the home (or other setting) strongly influence how far people are receptive to training. Considerable amounts of time, effort and resources are often needed to ensure that care staff, and the work setting, are open to learning.

From this it follows that

> 'different intervention strategies are needed based on careful assessment of the work setting and the standards of care being provided.'
> (Payne, 1991b).

All the work of this Programme—and much of the experience of the other CHI work too—underlines the importance of understanding the role of training in relation to the overall purposes, philosophy, history and management of the organisation as well as the particular home.

It seems probable that agendas for training which have been developed from the grassroots will expose weak management and splits in the staff groups. If people are asked about their needs—about the running of the home—their major preoccupations are likely to surface although not necessarily in an explicit way. If outsiders are involved in training events it is also likely that they—like consultants everywhere—will be vulnerable to being used by an unhappy staff group or by an anxious individual. This was certainly the experience of many consultants across the CHI: people attempted to draw them in to solve problems that were not being tackled internally.

The point that Payne underlines is that training can, too easily, be 'plugged in' as a way of attempting to deal with something that is really a management responsibility. This leads us to suggest that the audit should identify management implications and that this stage should involve senior levels in considering the wider issues before a training programme is devised. There is a danger otherwise that the training agenda could be used to address management issues or fudge fundamental problems relating to policy, resources or priorities.

The planning and management of change are, therefore, an issue for training. What role does training play? Payne's question 'Is development the key to effective training?' —might be reversed. Is training the key to development—to responding to changing demands and a changing environment? We saw that it was the policy of several of the project agencies to use training approaches to move care homes forward. Meeting inspection criteria and quality standards were part of the motivation but the implications of the trend to include residents in quality review were also recognised. To meet residents' demands requires staff and management to be responsive and flexible, to adapt, acquire new skills and knowledge. Training approaches have a part to play in ensuring that people are open to change and able to make responses without losing the integrity and continuity of service.

One of the issues which the Programme experience raises is how far training needs can and should be developed and understood at grassroots in relation to the individual establishment and how far these have to be defined in relation to more strategic objectives. One of the implications is that in-house review opens up the possibility of new perspectives and new priorities which may either implicitly or explicitly, challenge traditional notions and top-down expectations and requirements. If this is so, then a further implication for management is that of understanding the shifts and trends which are taking place in relation to user demands and expectations within establishments on the one hand and balancing these against top-down and strategic requirements on the other.

Although we noted that creating the kind of climate in which staff can be responsive to training opportunities is mainly a local issue and one which is determined strongly by the head of the establishment, there are also implications here for the role of senior managers. What kind of signals does the home manager require in order to create a more open culture both between staff and between staff and residents? What kind of discretion does a staff group require in order to respond to local needs and demands? The experience of the projects was that training cultures and approaches to providing staff development opportunities—the culture and climate of staff development—do have to be supported by a management approach which is based in the same values and assumptions if they are to be successful. We would argue that training and staff development are an intrinsic element of service provision and, therefore, an essential part of the overall task of management.

Overview

THE CHI: A COHERENT PROGRAMME FOR QUALITY SERVICE?

There are several questions to be asked about the connection between the Programmes and the materials they produced:

- are the approaches compatible?

- can they be integrated in practice?

- does CHI represent a comprehensive approach to ensuring quality of service?

Are the CHI Materials Compatible?

The answer to this must be 'yes' in principle. The results of the project work and the way these were formulated into practice guides show clear similarities based in shared values and assumptions about the promotion of quality and about how to pursue change and development:

- quality of the resident's life is the central goal;

- development work relies on stimulating ideas and changing attitudes both inside and outside homes;

- the home must be seen as a whole: any agenda for change has to relate to the purposes and objectives of the individual establishment;

- the status and training of staff is central;

- processes of change must involve users—in defining the direction of, and priorities for, service development, in setting standards and assuring quality;

- the aims of a new approach must be owned by those who have to implement or develop new ideas/ways of doing things;

- changes at the grassroots require the support of the organisation;

- quality is a collective responsibility: of a staff team not any one individual; of management not only the head of a home; of users and their families.

150

In these ways the CHI materials show an underlying compatibility broadly stemming from a commitment to residents' interests and the value of the contribution of frontline managers and staff. Some of these aspects will be discussed in more detail in Chapter 7 when we look at the issues to emerge across the Initiative.

Is the Integration of CHI Approaches a Practicality?
The Programmes were not able to plan integrated projects but experience indicated that, whatever the prime focus of the project, other aspects of running the home were likely to enter the discussions and become important in planning the work. Project consultants in particular commented that it was difficult, and sometimes obstructive in practice, to make clear separation between different areas of work.

Work in some establishments led quite straightforwardly to work which was the direct concern of another Programme. For example, a number of establishments involved in training projects identified a need to clarify the purposes of the home and to review aims and objectives. Staff involved in discussing and writing up accounts of the establishment became aware of the importance of involving residents. In at least one case this led to the development of a type of quality group on the lines of the IQA model. Others decided to carry out an IQA review. In several cases reviewing the work of the home prompted thought about the importance of producing good information about the home for current and potential residents.

Equally, some homes involved in the IQA trial recognised the implications for staff practice and development which emerged from the review: the kind of training needs identified included those relating to handling complaints, creating opportunities for residents' participation and consultation, residents' activities, the provision and exchange of information.

These observations—particularly those from projects which tried out materials from more than one Programme—indicate that the different approaches can be integrated in practice.

First, the models described by the Programmes and the tools developed for pursuing change are very similar. Three Programmes advocated some form of reflective stock-taking of the current situation and each underlined the importance of considering the home as a whole. Decisions about what might require change then followed. The task for the home was to decide which issues to tackle first and how.

Second, the manuals and guidelines were designed to be adaptable. The degree of adaptability related to the extent to which managers and staff were guided in thinking about the issues in relation to their establishment. Manuals or practice guides which promote further thought and refinement ensure that any action taken is relevant and in line with local purposes and resources. Those which provide blueprints for action or prescribe specific programmes were less useful and harder to adapt.

Third, issues which require attention may be identified in a number of different ways. Any or all of the materials could lead to the same kind of conclusion about what needs to be improved or changed: any could, potentially, prompt thought about other aspects of providing quality care. Looked at from the perspective of the home the areas of work were not distinct but overlapped and influenced each other.

There were indications, too, of the issues which could lead to some difficulties in using two or more of the materials together. However, some of these are circumstances that would make the implementation of any change or development problematic:

- conflicting objectives between innovation and the existing aims of the establishment;

- the work demanded significant change in the working approaches or attitudes of staff;

- different approaches used materials which were difficult to operate at the same time;

- work required different time scales;

- competition for resources;

- variable attractiveness to staff, users, officers, agency, residents.

Is the CHI a Comprehensive Approach to Ensuring Quality?
In order to provide residential accommodation and services all care homes carry out a similar range of functions. These are implied by the Wagner recommendations and many were the focus of CHI work. The obvious gaps were any direct focus on financial or resource management, on management or on administration: aspects which were not directly referred to in the Wagner review but which underlie the decision making and action implied in implementing the CHI materials. The pursuit of quality relies on a coherence between the way these functions are carried out and complement each other.

If we take the functions carried out by the care establishment one by one we can log which aspects are tackled, at least to some extent, by CHI work. Table 6.1 gives a resumé of Programme coverage of the main functional areas.

TABLE 6.1

Care Home Function	Aspects Addressed by CHI Programmes
1. Establishing a coherent set of aims and a working philosophy for the home	CESSA, NISW and SCA materials all refer to the importance of clarifying aims and purposes for workers, residents and outsiders
2. Establishing effective management and administration	None of the Programmes addressed management directly but the work demonstrated the value of clear working relationships, reliable support and efficient administration
3. Establishing a secure living and working environment: contracts and clear expectations for staff and residents	CESSA: aspects of residents' rights and security NISW: aspects of staff needs PSI *Home Truths*: information exchange
4. Establishing resources for appropriate physical, social and emotional needs of residents, including security of finance and tenure	CESSA and SCA: residents' social and emotional needs CESSA: residents' values PSI *Home Truths*: information relating to long-term security
5. Establishing the identity and relationships of the home: within the agency, within the local community, with the families and carers of residents, with potential users	SCA: links and external relationships between the home, residents and local communities PSI: informing people about services CESSA: involvement of relatives and other outsiders
6. Maintaining the physical environment: buildings, furnishings and fabric	CESSA: focused questions on the physical environment
7. Direct provision of services and care	CESSA: residents, staff and outsiders comment on all aspects of the home NISW, SCA audit of home and its services
8. Staffing: recruitment, training, staff support and development	NISW: staff training needs and preparing training plans
9. Setting standards and ensuring quality	CESSA review, NISW and SCA audits address quality measures

Between them the Programmes addressed a number of the functions implied in running a care establishment. However, this does not add up to a comprehensive series of manuals and guides. There are gaps across the functions and within each functional area. It is better to see the CHI work as a series of related approaches which overlap to some extent but which do appear to prompt people to think in similar or parallel ways about how the functions inter-relate. This convergence may well stem from the emphasis they place on the resident as a source of information and critical comment.

The CHI experience shows that a lack of coherence or complementarity between functional areas, either within the home or in the wider organisation, often lies behind difficulties in achieving high standards: this we discuss in Part Three.

PART THREE

Learning from the Caring in Homes Initiative

Chapter 7

THE RESIDENTIAL EXPERIENCE

So far we have discussed the work of the CHI Programme by Programme. As we have seen, the projects which they ran aimed to bring about benefits for residents and in a variety of ways. In the previous chapters we discussed the results and the potential usefulness of the Programmes' work.

In this chapter we move on to consider general themes and issues that emerged and the lessons to be drawn from the Initiative as a whole. There are, of course, a number of important perspectives which we could pursue but, to preserve focus, our organising frame has been to consider what is revealed about the experience of people living and working in residential establishments, to look at the implications of these for practice and management and to ask how far the Programmes help to ensure that resident interests are understood and met.

First we consider what, if any, new perspectives have emerged about the needs, expectations and priorities of people living in establishments and how these are met. What contribution does the CHI work make to addressing the issues raised?

Second, the experience of living in residential establishments is intimately connected with the working lives of the staff and the relationships between them and residents. In many ways the staff too are consumers of the residential experience. We look, therefore, at the issues which emerged concerning staff interests, their work and the way they approach care practice.

In the next chapter we look at the issues raised by these discussions as they relate to the quality of residents' lives, and help to identify the kind of changes that are implied in establishments and organisations.

Learning about the Experience of Residents

In Chapter 2 we identified some of the main issues for residential provision from interviews we conducted during the first phase of the Initiative. We noted that there were a number of shared concerns and, on the whole, similar perceptions about future needs and trends across the care groups. A central issue for the evaluation was to understand more about the needs, wishes and experience of residents, how these are articulated and responded to.

The Wagner review set an important precedent in looking at all the main care groups. The importance of this is, perhaps, only just beginning to be fully appreciated and the work of the Initiative certainly endorses the value of taking a generic approach.

Working across the groupings highlighted how assumptions and established notions about care needs are changing and can be challenged. Some of the major resistances to development came from the way management, professionals and care staff viewed their role, from a lack of clarity about what an establishment was trying to achieve and a failure to recognise what is of most importance to residents.

One of the key issues to emerge was that there are important areas of common cause which outweigh some of the distinctions which are assumed to exist between the interests and needs of different care groups. With this in mind we have chosen to organise our discussion around generic points rather than address residents' interests group by group as we did earlier.

Addressing the groupings as if their need for services were fundamentally different tends to perpetuate stereotypical ideas and responses and serves the interests of providers, practitioners and various professionals rather than those of the user. Generally, care is organised to meet special needs but we found that categorising people in this way can prevent service providers from recognising and responding to ordinary needs.

What issues emerged from the projects concerning the way residents' interests are voiced, understood and responded to?

A general finding was that the majority of the residents with whom we talked or spent time in the course of visiting homes were experiencing restrictions, difficulties and frustrations that represented an erosion of their rights as citizens and fell short of a reasonable quality of life. What is important, we believe, about our observations is that the reasons for people's lack of comfort or contentment appeared to be associated with broadly similar issues.

The difficulties expressed were, in nearly every case, related to weak social and emotional ties, poor or troubled family links, lack of friendships and other social contacts and a general absence of feeling valued and special. Many people lacked opportunities to be purposeful, productive or active and to plan for the next stage of their life. Linked with these issues were those relating to the need for a sense of security and control over their affairs. The experience of moving into a residential establishment is, however welcome, always a time of great change and upheaval: unresolved feelings of loss and dislocation are often the cause of continuing unhappiness. (See, for example, Lowden 1992.) Elderly people, in particular saw themselves as 'being of no use to anyone': they valued opportunities, however small, for reciprocating help recieved from others.

The importance of the physical environment was, of course, very evident and endorsed by everyone with whom we spoke. The way that space can open up or confine social contacts, the difference between self-chosen decorations and all-over-the-same pale green, the misery of unreliable plumbing, the significance of fresh paint and flowers ... the importance of such things was emphasised again and again. Even so, some of the importance stems from their symbolic value in showing respect and an accurate awareness of needs of the people living and working in a home.

Often, it seemed that people were talking about the shortcomings of physical care or the environment of the home as a way of indicating that they felt depersonalised or unspecial. The problem with poor laundry marking, for example, is not only that you may lose your own clothes and end up with someone else's but that it is another indication that you have lost part of your identity and are not regarded by others. Although the reasons for a resident's sense of isolation may often lie in their past or in current family relationships—that is, not directly with the way things are run in the establishment—it is, nonetheless, relevant to ask what responsibility staff and management, together with residents themselves and their relatives, should take in addressing such distress.

Focus on social integration needs

One way of understanding this picture is to make an analytical distinction between physical and material needs on the one hand and social and emotional needs on the other. Maslow (1954) suggested that human needs could be understood as a hierarchy. Using a modified version of this model, Faulk (1988) refers to basic material resource needs— physiological, physical safety and security—underpinning more complex needs for social integration—for love and belonging, for self-esteem and for growth and fulfilment. He found that the various aspects of social integration were highly important to people in the residential establishments he studied and that meeting these needs contributed most significantly to their quality of life. Adequate provision for physical and resource needs was appreciated but meeting social and emotional needs were valued more than high standards in the physical environment. This was endorsed from an analysis of our data base: standards of care were judged less in terms of physical resources than by the quality of relationships and general climate of the place.

We are not suggesting that this distinction is in any sense possible or real in practice—human needs and experience do not fall neatly into categories of this sort—but it does provide a useful way of considering CHI findings.

In focusing on the social integration needs and the emotional and social experience of residents, we are attempting to highlight and provide an account of what came across, not only to us as evaluators, but also to other outsiders involved in the projects—such as IQA interviewers and Programme consultants. These observations raise important issues and so, in taking a resident-centred point of view, we concentrate on the messages we received about social and emotional needs rather more than physical ones.

Focus on individualised rather than collective, group-based needs

A significant consequence of highlighting social integration is that it places more emphasis on the individual resident than on aggregated or collective needs. Typically, however, services are organised around the needs of particular groups or categories and there have been good reasons for this. There are patterns to the way people require support and services and these do tend to cluster around age and ability. One way of ensuring that such needs are responded to is to group together professionals and practitioners with relevant knowledge, skills and equipment in a more or less specialised setting.

However, this can lead to significant difficulties in meeting individual needs. The CHI projects revealed some of the practical, organisational and attitudinal difficulties to be addressed in meeting individual, idiosyncratic preferences in a group-based setting. The issues are complex in that they involve mediating and balancing between individual and group, and between different interests. Nearly all care homes specialise for particular groups of people and cater for them on a segregated basis: collective rather than individual needs are highlighted.

We discuss some of the aspects of policy, provision and care practice that influence the way in which residents' needs are recognised and met. We consider the implications of these and the extent to which the work of the Initiative shows a way ahead.

Residents as Whole People

A fundamental principle of all care provision is that people's rights are preserved and one of the bases of ensuring good practice is to consider each person as having a set of rights as a citizen and as an individual. To think in terms of care groupings is to think of a type of resident—a category of person. The label describes some, but by no means all, or even the most important, of the characteristics of those who belong to that group. Labelling of this kind is a way in which others note—and give precedence to—particular features and respond according to their own ideas. Discrimination based on colour or race or age are obvious examples.

Across the care groups individuals tend to be defined by the setting or home they enter. The SCA work showed how neighbours can stigmatise residents of a care establishment if people are not known as individuals but seen as a type of person. There were numerous examples of elders who lost confidence and self motivation on entering a home because they adapted to the dominant culture—often one that assumed greater dependence and frailty than was necessary. These are familiar examples to anyone working in the residential field. The issue seems to be that people can be defined, provided for and their needs understood in relation to only one part of their total personality. It is easy to see the dominant problems associated with disablement, with being elderly and frail, with being the victim of abuse, with alcohol misuse, but these can become overdetermining.

A further problem is that, in attending to specific needs, collective provision tends to emphasise parts of people—the disabled part, the elderly part, the sick part, the alcoholic part—rather than whole person-alities. The whole person is lost sight of and assumptions are made about the individual on the basis of a collective stereotype.

But there was plenty of evidence from which to challenge the collective stereotypes. Our quotes are mainly from staff although most were well aware of the shortcomings of thinking in categorical terms.

The kind of comments that were made are illustrated:

Of elders:

'All they want to do is sit ... we've tried to interest them in doing things.'
'Elderly people can't do much.'
'The people here are too frail to get out.'
'She always sits there like that, she doesn't want to be bothered.'

But the majority of elders we met revealed how isolated or lonely they felt. There were so many who wanted company but did not know how to reach out to other people. One of the most common comments from the IQA interviews was that staff were friendly and very caring but too busy to spend time talking. Several IQA interviewers told us of their distress because the residents so much wanted their company and to talk. Whereas physical isolation tended to be recognised by staff, social isolation was rarely noticed—how can you be lonely in a care home?

Of people with drug problems:

'The problem with drug abusers is they can be very unreliable.'

But an SCA project showed how well local people responded to the opportunity to be helped by residents from a local hostel.

Of people with learning disabilities:

'People with a learning disability need to be protected.'
'They need a lot of guidance and help.'
'They can embarass people when they are out—then the home's reputation suffers.'

But residents told us that they wanted to be allowed to take risks and organise their own affairs. Projects showed how, with appropriate help, residents were able to make their own radio broadcast, enjoy outings to the pub, take measured risks with complicated transport systems, contribute to making an information video.

Of children:

'Youngsters have to be able to get out and play...'
'We have responsibility for children ... a parental role.'

But adults with disabilities and older people need to play and be active too. In one home the level of mobility increased significantly once it was realised that there was a traffic jam problem with zimmers and wheel-chairs. In another, people moved about much more when they had the opportunity to use the garden and visit friends in other parts of the building.

Staff have responsibilities for adults as well as children: although the nature of that responsibility is different and shared with the resident.

The following extract from a CCETSW guide lists skills needed by staff in residential child care (CCETSW 1992). But these are equally relevant for work with other groups of residents—for example, isolated elders:

'• handling dependent relationships

• helping (children) to feel valued and important both individu-ally and in the group

• helping (children) to feel loved and genuinely cared for

• handling issues of sexuality, intimacy and physical contact (in child care)

• developing (childrens') enthusiasms and interests and provid-ing appropriate cultural opportunities

• learning details of family support and other outreach work, of helping (children) to manage family and friendship relationships and (where necessary) to cope with the denial or loss of contact

• coping with ambiguity, differences, uncertainty.'

(CCETSW,1992)

This can be read as a generic statement about the skills needed to provide a living base for anyone in residence. The detailed attention to the emotional and social needs of children is based in the assumption that staff take a parental responsibility which is not seen as relevant or appropriate for adults. This is, of course, valid but there are parallel responsibilities which staff might recognise in relation to other care groups. Our evidence is that the inertia or apparent helplessness of some adult residents is, in many cases, a quickly learned response to a climate of 'total care' where staff do the work, make the decisions, set the pattern of day-to-day living. There is instead, it can be argued, a role for staff in helping people to retain or to realise their power to act, to make decisions, to speak out for what they want. Just as children need support and the right environment to help them with the business of growing up and forming an identity, so anyone in a group-living situation needs opportunities to preserve or establish their individual path.

Traditional client or care group categorisations have been helpful in recognising special needs and marshalling expertise, facilities and resources to meet them. Specialised homes have been the norm and will continue to be needed. But the work of the different CHI Programmes prompts thought about the bases of people's need for residential services. Should these be understood in terms of physical or age-related needs—or social needs or preferences? Again the theme is the importance of seeing people as individuals rather than categories.

The following vignettes are true of a variety of different people and do not particularly relate to their age or ability. They represent the views of people we met during the research and they serve to demonstrate a different way of thinking about people who require either accommodation or services or both.

A positive choice
We met many people whose first choice was to live with others in a residential home. For them a care home was not a last resort or somewhere they had to be because there were no alternatives: they wanted the company and reassurance of living with others. They were actively seeking the benefits of a group setting: belonging, sharing with others, being securely looked after. People in this category included young children who felt safer 'in care' than at home; older people who no longer wanted the responsibilities of living alone; people with mental health problems who preferred the company of people like themselves and who found group living a freedom from family tensions; people moving on from a long period in hospital or other large institution. Thus, for many people finding security, company and understanding outweighed the limitations. The underlying issue is that people usually—though not always—compare their current situation with a previous living arrangement. People in this category were those who had found the place they wanted to be—certainly for the foreseeable future.

A way forward
There were also people who valued residential care because it provided an opportunity for personal change—like physical rehabilitation, mental healing or growing up—or which allowed them time to make new arrangements. People were looking for a particular kind of transitional

home—a place that would provide help and support while they gained or regained skills, confidence or secured practical resources. Many people enter residential establishments with the expectation of moving to a more independent situation in time. These expectations were equally true for an elderly person recovering from a fall after a period in hospital, a young adult with learning disabilities who had been living with parents, a person with alcohol problems, someone who had been in a long-term psychiatric ward and an older teenager in care. These were people who wanted to move on but equally required support and time to do so.

Not their choice

There were those for whom living in a residential establishment was not their choice. Such people had resisted, and continued to resent, being away from their own locality or having to change their lifestyle: some had come to accept their circumstances but many were preoccupied by their plight. People in this position included a young man who felt co-erced into following a therapeutic regime, a man in his sixties in a home with much older and very frail people, an elderly woman who could not accept that her son-in-law could not provide her with a home after her daughter's death. For each there was a legitimate reason for the move into a home but these related more to the needs of their families than themselves: they were not reconciled to their situation.

It is a matter of grave concern that most of the people we met—informally and in more formal discussions—came into this last category, irrespective of age, ability or length of time in the establishment. The homes in which we met these residents were not out of the ordinary. The majority of places we visited throughout the research were pleasant enough, well furnished, apparently comfortable and cheerful places. The problem lay, in the majority of cases, not in the fabric of the homes but with a lack of awareness of the individual resident's feelings, needs and wishes for their life. Their social integration needs were either not understood or people did not have access to the means of meeting them. Some recognition— some opportunity to talk about their distress, as they did to us as researchers—could have gone some way to helping people in such circumstances feel less rejected or powerless.

People's reasons for seeking or avoiding collective living are related to individual history, to personal preference, to family relationships and social circumstances, to financial means and the availability or absence of real alternatives. We suggest that it is more helpful to consider people in residential establishments not by their age, physical or mental ability but according to their experience, expectations and aspirations for the future. What these vignettes helped us to see is that the points of reference for judging the quality and relevance of a particular form of accommodation or service lie with the user/resident/individual. The essential judgements both about the suitability of residential care and about the kind of accommodation and services and the lifestyle that these afford are, in good part, subjective and can only be articulated in reference to the experience and expectations of the individual.

In what ways did the CHI research show how these needs can be recognised and met?
The CHI guides place some emphasis on resident interests and the means by which these can be identified.

The work of IQA showed that people—staff as well as residents—may need help in order to voice their ideas, preferences or difficulties. The formation of a specific group and talking to an outsider in a fairly structured way did provide people with an opportunity to speak about themselves. The benefits of speaking out lay not only in what was said. A valuable spin off was that people also had the experience of being taken seriously and participating in the life of the home. These affirmed belonging and self-worth. The trial projects indicated that running a review that included people was a way of establishing a greater climate of openness in which it was easier for people to share and exchange views.

The work on training showed how staff were able to develop greater sensitivity to the needs of residents and to appreciate how ideas, priorities and ways of looking at life in the home might differ between residents and between staff and residents. Again it seemed that the issue was one of opening up new perspectives and possibilities for dialogue.

The emphasis of Window in Homes projects was on social contacts and creating opportunities for residents both inside the establishment and in the community. Highlighting the importance of social integration parallels these concerns. Many of the projects involved staff in reaching out beyond the boundaries of the home. They were making contacts with a variety of people and agencies that they would not, perhaps, have done otherwise. One of the questions that this work raises is the extent to which workers based in residential establishments should be reviewing their practice to include, for example, networking, forms of community action or liaison with leisure and educational services. Finding or creating opportunities for residents does require active preparation and negotiation with outsiders as well as supporting residents in taking their own steps.

The PSI publication *Home Truths* looked at the importance of an exchange of information at the point of entry. The checklists emphasised physical needs but did miss an opportunity to focus on aspects of social and emotional needs and future wishes.

Meeting Individual Needs in a Group Setting
Traditionally residential provision has been organised on the assumption that, in meeting the needs which define the care group, the most significant problems facing the individual will be catered for.

The fact that there are limits to meeting the needs of the individual in a group care setting is well recognised by managers and care staff and frequently discussed in care settings. However, the experience of the projects suggests that there are a number of ways to create a better balance.

What has to be provided on a collective basis?

There is room for reviewing which aspects of accommodation and service have to be organised on a collective basis and which can be made more user specific. We saw how new ideas about organising meals made a considerable difference to individual choice about when to get up or go to bed, about what to eat, with whom and where. Traditionally meals are communal and organised around the cook's hours but for many flexibility is highly valued. Using a breakfast bar, having the alternative of cold meals, 'phoning the local dial-a-meal, using micro-waves—each brings the possibility of variety and independence of institutional norms.

Some homes were looking at the use of private and communal space to find ways of allowing greater flexibility. Others were involving residents in designing menus and children's homes were moving way from bulk purchasing in order to give young people experience of shopping, budgeting for and preparing meals. Could arrangements for bathing, room decoration, laundry, visits and social outings be equally flexible?

Recognition of social integration needs

One problem is that, up until now, services generally have placed more emphasis on, and have been better equipped to understand, how to meet people's physical and age related needs—the basis on which people are categorised and assumed to be the same. But this has meant that rather less attention has been given to their social and emotional needs—the bases on which people tend to be different and to express a variety of preferences and ideas which do not necessarily relate to age or ability. We found nothing to indicate that social and emotional needs were more important to one group than another. In one home, for example, awareness that someone was taking a special interest seemed to result in one or two people with mental frailty wandering less and showing less confusion. Guidance on child care practice and training lays emphasis on understanding the importance of family but we know that family ties (whether present or lost) vitally affect everyone's sense of wellbeing. Listening to a woman of over ninety talking about her mother and how she misses her was poignant and powerful in making the point.

One issue that was infrequently mentioned by residents—in the IQA interviews or in our contacts—was that of intimate relationships. One exception was that younger residents with physical disabilities were able to use an IQA review to express frustration at the lack of opportunity to form and enjoy sexual and other close relationships: staff were surprised and upset at their own lack of awareness. Staff in some establishments for youngsters and younger adults did talk about the sexual and other relationship needs of the residents but this was often in the context of how to supervise contacts and protect, rather than provide opportunities for forming and fulfilling friendships. Residents and staff in homes for older people rarely mentioned such things. While this is not surprising, it is an indication that, according to the age of the resident, close friendships and sexual fulfilment tend to be seen either as a problem or irrelevant!

An ordinary life is about managing personal relationships, trying to succeed at snooker, worrying about work and money. Painful or not, they are the aspects of life which create a sense of self and identity, difference and self-worth. The means of ensuring that people have the opportunity to lead fulfilled lives lies in supporting the growth or maintainance of all aspects of life: physical activities, employment, leisure, personal relationships and social contacts. These are the ingredients of life that help to make the difference between isolation and boredom and a life with a purpose and a future.

On a practical level, people in care homes are often cut off from the means of making or maintaining links. For many elders, for example, making a phone call was almost impossible. In principle, they might have been able to use the public 'phone in the corridor or in the staff room but making and receiving calls was then a public rather than a private activity. The sense of being cut off from the means of reaching important people and arranging one's own affairs was a major cause of people feeling isolated.

Recognition of personal history and the importance of the future

What also tends to happen is that people are assessed for or seek residential care at a particular point in their life. For the majority of elderly people—entering from their home or from hospital—this happens in a hurry, often in an atmosphere of crisis and with little time to prepare. Except for the very young this tends to freeze the frame of reference in the present: people are known for who they are now while their personal history and links with the past can easily get lost.

The importance of social and cultural networks is increasingly understood in relation to patterns of caring and these have featured in studies of informal care in the community (Wenger, 1984; Abrams et al, 1989; Bulmer 1987). What is less well appreciated is their importance in relation to the well being of the individual. A number of projects provided insights into the importance of social and family connections. Those involving black and ethnic minority groups endorsed the signficance of maintaining racial and cultural links: where such ties were lost or were disregarded or inadequately understood, people felt particularly isolated and discriminated against.

One of the most telling aspects in understanding the experience of residents across the care groups was the extent to which they held a positive view of the future. Again, this tends to differ markedly across care groups. For example, there is always a strong future orientation in planning for children in care but this is rarely the case for people with long-term mental health problems or those who are elderly. Yet planning ahead is crucial for elders. These are people who may not have much longer in which to arrange their affairs. How many care plans cover someone's wishes for their funeral, for the disposition of their precious things? Social integration is about saying goodbye and preparing for endings as well as planning new opportunities: it is about severing links as well as creating them.

Care plans help to identify needs but they do not meet them
Care plans were widely valued as a way of identifying individual needs and planning. They were seen as an important means of ensuring that staff knew about individual plans and that there was a continuity of approach. However, there was a tendency to leave it at that. The existence of a plan is not the same as its active pursuit. Equally, care planning can become a rather stereotyped affair following a series of questions on a pro forma that does little to challenge what is or is not happening or to prompt new ideas or aspirations. Involving the resident in the planning was generally accepted as good practice although we found a number of homes that did not do so. But if planning is not matched by an awareness of what the plan means in terms of everyday opportunities and relationships, it is only an administrative exercise from the resident's point of view. Talking day by day with a resident as ideas occur, as issues arise, might be more effective than formalised, written plans. We talked to a number of people who rejected formal care plans on this basis.

The care home does not have to do it all
Traditionally care homes have been seen as places providing total care. The home set out—and was expected—to provide for all the needs of the residents and, in that respect, to be a self-sufficient living unit. We spoke earlier of how care establishments have been seen as places apart and the problems of isolation and misunderanding that this can bring. The other side of this is that the management can take on an all embracing responsibility for providing care that may be unnecessary and unwanted. For example, bringing a mini-shop or a hairdresser on site may be convenient, but does this mean people are less likely to go out—or be enabled to get out and about—to use local facilities and talk to local people? We saw that bringing an advocate in to help facilitate a resident group had great value but equally it might have been even more beneficial for the residents to go outside the establishment for such support.

Relatives, friends, partners and workmates make up the social fabric of a normal life. Are there ways in which they could be more involved in the life of a resident? Again, attention is paid to the family ties of children in residential establishments: social workers and care staff are expected to be active in ensuring, for example, that a child's important relationships are preserved, that an appropriate placement is found. Why not give as much attention to all care groups?

The isolation of elders, for example, cannot be fully explained by an absence of family or an unwillingness to make new contacts. A survey of elderly people in day and residential care, carried out by Counsel and Care (1991), showed that only 16% had no family who could visit whereas 40% were either not visited or had visits once a month or less. The majority (82%) said they would welcome visits from volunteers but only 34% received such visits. There is, on this evidence, room for establishments to take an active role in fostering contacts for residents and encouraging personal links.

How far did the work of CHI projects help to address issues relating to individualisation?

The issue underpinning individualisation is that of difference. Any approach to care practice and service provision that helps to value and appreciate the differences between people will enhance opportunities for their self fulfilment.

The work of IQA was founded on a recognition that people living in residential homes, their relatives and carers and the staff working in them have different needs and interests. Much of the developmental work was concerned with establishing ways to ensure that the review incorporated and reflected this range of interests and that these were considered in making decisions about action. Although the system does not set out to review individual needs directly, it does establish the value of each person's views. The importance of involving relatives was highlighted by the IQA work and although it did not develop a full debate about the potential role that they can play, it has helped to put them on the map. It is close family and friends who know the resident well and who can help them to establish the lifestyle they prefer.

The work of the training programme did not address issues relating to the needs of the individual directly but the overall approach was to promote shared learning by valuing the working experience and knowledge of the staff.

By emphasising the importance of the links people have outside the home in the local community, the Window in Homes work also helped to focus attention on the kind of contacts that residents value and how these might be established. It showed that thinking about social needs in terms of collective outings or in-house bingo sessions has its place but does not go far in meeting the need of the individual for their special relationships and links.

The PSI work pointed to the different ways in which individual choice can be promoted—by providing information for service users and by obtaining relevant information about the individual.

Professional Interests and Residents' Needs

Professional interests have tended to dominate the way services are designed, offered and reviewed. We noted earlier that people are labelled in terms of their physical and mental abilities or age-related needs— categories which have grown up around medical and other areas of professional expertise. In the first part of the book we referred to the interests of those who work in the field of social and care services and how professional identity, status and career prospects may be closely linked to the different care categories.

This has meant that services have, typically, been designed around areas of professional knowledge. As a corollary, people have been assessed for services according to whether they meet the eligibility criteria set by those who run the service. Service development has thus been strongly influenced by the ideas and assumptions of professionals and practitioners.

This may shift with emphasis on needs-led, individual assessment for care services in the community and the split between purchasers and providers, but there will remain considerable professional interest in preserving areas of expertise, employment and career advancement and these can easily mask, or be in tension with, residents' needs. One mental health agency involved in a project, with a nursing and hospital-based background, is unlikely to move very fast towards greater user involvement and participation in the running of its hostels and homes. This would not only overturn years of history during which residents were seen—and continue to be seen—as dependent patients who need round the clock supervision. It would also require a different regime, different skills and knowledge leading to a new kind of staff appointment that was no longer based in traditional nursing or hospital practice.

There is certainly resistance from people involved in running nursing homes to the idea of ending the distinction between care and nursing homes. But the difference between them is often hard to perceive and is becoming harder to justify. We saw a number of instances where the high level dependency of very frail people, for example, was being successfully met by care homes with support from community nurses and supportive GPs. The management and staff of these care homes were committed to their residents and could see no reason for them to go through the trauma of a move when their health deteriorated. They were dismissive of the idea that people needed any more special nursing or facilities than were available from ordinary community services. From a resident's point of view it is hard to disagree with them.

These examples give a glimpse of the kind of shifts in attitude or service structure that might be implied in taking a more resident-led approach to service development. In the interests of individual rights and good practice, residents should shape provision not other way round. This implies greater flexibility of provision and a high degree of resident involvement both at an individual and at a collective level. It is also in line with the intentions of community care arrangements for individual care planning.

Do the CHI approaches have the potential to challenge professional interests?

The CHI projects, apart from those addressing information provision, were not working at the level of a service as a whole and were not addressing aspects of organisational development. The grassroots, in-house nature of the work meant that it was unlikely to influence strategic thinking directly. However, the values embraced by the Programmes and the approaches they used did raise questions about traditional ways of looking at services and how they are developed. The representation of interests on an IQA Quality Group, for example, allows for the possibility that resident and lay views might differ from those of the management and staff. The involvement of basic-level care workers in defining a training plan for the home is a signal that their views are valid and may differ from those of senior managers.

There are many implications that flow from grassroots review and innovation: one is that it implicitly challenges top-down and established views. We will disuss this in more detail in relation to lessons that the CHI offers about initiating change.

Revising Notions of Care to be Consistent with Residents' Needs

The provision of residential services is based on ideas about the kind of help and support that people in residential settings require. There have, until recently, been two linked assumptions about residential care, which are being challenged:

- that people entering a home require total care and

- the establishment should provide all that a resident needs.

The Wagner review made an invaluable distinction between the provision of accommodation and of services. People enter an establishment for a variety of reasons—some more based in accommodation needs and some relating to physical or psychological care needs. Separating accommodation and services allows greater differentiation and flexibility in thinking about the requirements of residents and how to meet them.

A further principle, but one that is not so well established, is that a care home is part of the community and as such can draw on community-based services and other resources. Residents then have access to the opportunities and facilities that are available to anyone in the community.

It was clear, however, across the projects, that traditional ideas of providing total care do still exist and that there are a high number of homes where ordinary services and facilities are not accessible to or used by residents.

One of the issues that came to our attention was the tendency of committed, caring but anxious staff to overprotect residents. Over protection is only a short step away from control and restriction. For example, there were people who were actively discouraged from going out unsupervised because of the possibility of geting lost. There were people who pointed out that although they wanted help getting into the bath, they then wanted to be left on their own.

The underlying issue is that of developing a consistent service approach that matches the wishes and needs of residents as individuals and as a living group. Problems stem from a mismatch between the care provided and what is actually wanted or needed.

What is meant or understood by caring varies widely and is rarely defined. In the absence of a working philosophy and an approach to the work that is shared by a staff group, care workers and more senior staff come to rely on various assumptions about what they should be doing. Untrained care workers, usually the staff who have most contact with residents day by day, draw on their own experience and resources in approaching their work. Since the majority of basic-level staff are women it is not surprising that notions about caring draw heavily on child care and family experience.

There is a danger that such notions do not fit well with the needs of the residents either as a group or as individuals. Even where the fit is good there is a problem that, if assumptions about care practice are not discussed, they can become fixed and inappropriate over time.

Some of the ideas which individuals and staff groups held about caring are described briefly to show the range of different assumptions that are made about the care task. In doing so we are making no case about whether these models are right or wrong, good or bad in themselves: different approaches will fit different situations and—more importantly different individuals—at different times.

- *child care model:* this is based on a protective and parental role in relation to someone who is less powerful and more vulnerable. Such responses can easily be evoked by adults with disability or who are frail but these can be patronising and overprotective and lead to a serious erosion of peoples' rights. It is a set of assumptions that can be just as inappropriate for children and young people. Generally, it tends to act against self motivation, risk-taking, reaching out and gaining confidence. It can, however, be appropriate for a highly vulnerable person— the victim of abuse, for example—for a short period. To deny someone close emotional care for fear of their dependency can be as damaging as overprotection.

- *kinship model:* this is based on the way close relatives and other members of an extended family relate to and take responsibility for each other. It differs from other models in assuming a form to the relationships between residents and staff based in cultural rather than organisational norms. Thus, in a home run for Asian elders, the younger workers always deferred to their elders however frail: there was no question of treating them as dependent children or people unable to speak for themselves.

Notions of kinship relationships are obviously culturally determined and vary widely. But where these fit the cultural and religious background of the residents such a model can be highly relevant and very reassuring. We noted the high level of importance attached to the shared values in homes run by, for example, a religious organisation or an ethnic minority group. People were reassured that their beliefs and values were understood—by staff and fellow residents—and would be respected as in their own community. In this sense the kinship model can offer a coherent set of assumptions that can be shared by staff and residents alike.

• *democratic model:* here the practice is for residents and staff to discuss and make joint decisions about the running of the establishment: everyone is expected to take responsibility and participate. This tends to assume that the residents are adults but it can be adapted for establishments for children and young people. In ensuring involvement and expression of views it goes some way to addressing issues of how to balance individual and collective needs and wishes.

• *hotel or catering model:* a down-to-earth approach which assumes that adults need little more than housekeeping services, meals and a bit of understanding company. A good natured and experienced worker in a hostel for older people with long term mental health problems commented: 'I used to run a pub: its not so different—someone to talk to and regular food and keeping an eye that they're all right.'

• *nursing or ward model:* this model assumes that the establishment should be run along the lines of a hospital ward. The emphasis is on getting practical and routine tasks completed according to the daily routine. Residents become the objects of care and are expected to co-operate in keeping the regime running smoothly. Success is judged by efficient task completion and adherence to institutional norms rather than direct consideration of the comfort and wellbeing of the residents.

• *expert or treatment model:* this model assumes that the purposes of the establishment are pursued by people with special training. It emphasises those aspects of care that are related to a particular therapeutic or rehabilitative programme. It is easy for basic-level workers to underestimate their importance if they do not sufficiently understand their part in the overall experience offered to residents.

There are important issues running through these models about the nature of the relationship between worker and resident. There are two sets of assumptions which significantly influence the approach to care which is taken. The first concerns who has power and authority and the way these are exercised. The second relates to the age at which or circumstances in which someone is accepted as having reached—or conversely lost—self responsibility. The general point we make is that the notion of care underpinning staff practice and the culture of a home should be made explicit and should fit the real needs of individual residents and the group as a whole. The realities of who makes decisions about what are fundamental to the experience of residents and their ability to exercise choice.

There is much to be thought about here. A number of issues hinge on when people are considered able to take responsibility for themselves and this varies considerably across and within the care groupings according to traditions of provision, professional views and degrees of parental involvement.

In what ways do the CHI programmes help to address these issues?
Ensuring that practice is relevant and does fit the needs and wishes of residents requires review and checking rather than operating set routines based on fixed assumptions. What was good practice one day can go out of date remarkably quickly given resident turnover, changing facilities and social expectations.

As we have noted before, the work done by CESSA, NISW and SCA all advocated some form of review of current practice and all emphasised the importance of clear statements about the purpose of the home and its working approaches. Although the system did not address the question of the fit between care practice and resident needs, the IQA reviews revealed some interesting mismatches between what individual residents wanted and what staff felt was appropriate. Different attitudes to risk taking between staff and residents were revealed in some of the SCA projects. These kind of examples helped to raise questions about care practice and the assumptions on which this was based.

Entering the Residential Establishment Should be Based on a Shared Understanding Between Resident and Provider

The basis of a fulfilled life should be that resident and provider are both fully aware of what each can expect of the other. There are limitations to personal freedoms involved in group-based living and there are ways in which residential care can never provide a truly homely living base. These realities need not mean that there is no room for a contract of understanding between the people involved. However, there are a number of reasons why it may be difficult for the potential resident to participate fully in a decision to enter an establishment.

First, there are people who are legally too young or deemed to be too mentally disabled to take full responsibility for such a decision. This does not mean youngsters or people with learning disabilities, for example, cannot be involved in discussions or be helped to understand what is happening. The thrust of the Children Act 1989, after all, is about ensuring that the needs and wishes of young people are properly taken into account in any decisions taken about their care. This principle is equally valid for adults.

Second, there are people who require care mainly because they have no relatives who are able or willing to provide the care needed. There are ways in which the interests of people with significant care needs are in tension with those of their family and carers. What is important is that the rights and needs of people needing support and care are recognised as distinct from, and considered separately from, those who care for them. One of the difficulties is the guilt that relatives have to deal with when they cease to provide direct care for someone for whom they continue to care deeply about.

Third, there are situations where the structured or prescriptive nature of the regime might make it difficult for someone to exercise a choice. But given full knowledge and discussion of what the establishment is providing it is possible for people to decide whether or not to accept the opportunity on offer. The keys are good information and open discussion.

The relevance of CHI work
The work of the PSI particularly emphasised the need for information exchange and the detail required by and about elderly people entering an establishment. This is the time when people can acquire the knowledge that helps them to make an informed choice based on accurate and detailed information about the home, how it is run and what it might be like to live there. The time for clarifying expectations and ensuring that people have a realistic picture of the home may be limited at the point of entry. But the task of ensuring a shared understanding should be of continuing importance. If circumstances in the home change residents have the right to know what is going on and why, and time to comment, react and adjust. The review work of IQA and NISW revealed that staff as well as residents need a good understanding of the purpose of the home and how it is run.

Residents Have Responsibilities As Well As Rights
Residents have a responsibility for their own lives. There is a marked tendency, whatever the age of the person entering an establishment, for them to surrender autonomy. Partly this seems to reflect the total care culture of many homes. People moving in quickly come to realise that they are not expected to make decisions about certain things. For some this is welcome: the responsibility of running a house has become a worry and they want freedom from making decisions. But, controversially, we can question whether residents should give up responsibilities and whether, if

175

they do so, it is the task of the care home to take up those responsibilities for them. There are situations, catered for by legal arrangements, when the responsibility for managing someone's affairs is taken up by a nominated person. But there are subtle ways in which residents can be discouraged from exercising responsibility.

Where this matters most, perhaps, is for people who are moving on to more independent living. Planning and preparing for one's future can be scary and it can be easy for care staff to take over rather than support someone in having a go and maybe failing. In many places staff were uneasy about how much to protect residents and how far to push them to try new opportunities.

One of the issues seems to be, therefore, whether staff or the individual resident takes primary reponsibility for planning and thinking ahead, for what gets done and for what actually happens. Is this a matter for discussion or negotiation or is there a clear link between a person's rights and their responsibilities? The questions are valid for all the care groups: how they are resolved will vary to some extent.

Residents have both a right to be consulted about and a responsibility to participate in the running of the home as whole. The right to be consulted has been established fairly recently as residents and their relatives have protested against home closures. But the practice of involving the users and consumers of services is, as we discusssed at the beginning of the book, not yet well established in care provision.

The contribution of CHI
An underlying issue for many staff groups was understanding and managing risk. Responsibility for residents was keenly felt by care workers. Training events, IQA feedback meetings and staff looking at enhancing community links often included discussion about the balance between rights, responsibilities and risks (see Lane, 1993).

A central issue for CHI has been establishing residents' rights and opportunities to speak out. Although this is acknowledged as a basic right alongside the right to complain, projects highlighted how people do need support and a sympathetic climate in order to voice their views. Commenting—let alone complaining—is not straightforward. The training projects, which took residents' interest as central, did lead to increased staff awareness of their situation. One of the findings from the IQA work was that although the management might be convinced of the benefits, residents themselves were often less keen on taking responsibility for commenting on the home. Quality Groups sometimes lacked resident members because people were reluctant to participate. The IQA projects indicated the importance of providing structured opportunities for people to comment. Emphasising the responsibilities of residents could offer another perspective on the democratisation of care homes and user empowerment.

Learning about the Experience and Interests of Staff

Just as the projects highlighted some aspects of residents' experience, they also provided insights into the concerns and interests of care staff. We comment here on a series of points that seem to us to highlight some important perspectives on their needs and experience. In doing so we make no particular distinction between basic-level workers, senior staff and managers.

The messages from the Wagner review (Wagner, 1988) and, more recently the Howe report on staffing (Howe, 1992), were clear about the low morale and the generally low status accorded to those who work in residential homes. Our interviews and observations endorsed these messages. The situation of many basic-level workers is a cause for concern and not only because there are significant numbers of people working for extremely poor pay in conditions that, in some places, even fail to meet health and safety regulations. The equal concern is that these are the people who tend to have most contact with residents. How can a quality service be provided through disaffected or unhappy staff? How could any manager expect to provide good care on such a basis?

But the majority of staff we met were committed to their work, had a strong sense of loyalty to their residents and were broadly welcoming, if cautious, of ideas about how the job might be done better. Staff were sometimes resistant to change but this was related to their work circumstances, their relationship with management and how ideas about making changes were presented.

Staff in Residential Establishments Feel Isolated

One of the strongest messages we received was how isolated many staff in residential establishments feel. This was as true of senior care staff and managers as basic-level workers. Part of the evidence came from the way that officers in charge and staff teams reacted to the availability of the project consultants and ourselves as evaluators. We expected people to be wary of university researchers and cautious in their responses. In very many cases, however, the reverse was true. Discussions with CHI project consultants confirmed our own observations that, in a significant number of homes, staff were eager for external support and keen to use guidance that was not forthcoming from their own agency. CHI consultants encountered staff groups that wanted their help in solving problems that were outside the scope of the project, managers who wanted backing in seeking more internal support, staff who saw the projects as a means of communicating their difficulties to senior managers. The arrival of someone with external authority was an occasion for staff to bid for their time and help.

Throughout CHI, across all groupings, we noted how much people wanted outside recognition and valued the time and interest of the CHI agencies. We were surprised how willing managers and staff were to help with our evaluation, which meant, in all cases, finding extra time for interviews and meetings, often on top of the project work.

Although enthusiasm for outside support can be taken as positive, it does signal problems in the present systems. It suggests that there are agencies where a lack of leadership, internal support, and effective management are adding to the isolation of care homes and are a significant cause of the low morale of workers.

Staff are Affected if the Purposes and Working Philosophy of the Establishment are not Clear

The observation that the aims and purposes of an establishment need to be clear may seem obvious but across the care groups we found a number of examples where project work revealed a lack of clarity about the detailed aims and the working philosophy of the home. Broad statements like 'to provide a home for people with learning disabilities' do not help much when a staff member is faced with an upset parent because their son has gone out *with* permission from the home and got drunk.

There are a number of difficulties that can follow from lack of clarity and absence of shared understanding about the job.

People in the same work group may not always understand each other if they are working on different assumptions about how to do the job. The earlier discussion about how people form their own notion about the kind of care that is needed links here: in the absence of a stated philosophy that is understood by everyone working in the home, workers will work to their own assumptions. There is, then, room for people to come to rather different conclusions about the work. Tensions between colleagues and different factions in staff groups were quite frequently revealed in the course of CHI projects. The wastage of time and energy that results from such difficulties and the cost in terms of personal stress can be considerable. Staff morale is obviously affected by any uncertainty about the work or relationships between colleagues.

Second, people were not necessarily clear about the kind of relationship that they should have with residents. All residents appreciate consistency in the way they are treated but for some this is particularly important. In providing child care, for example, or a safe place for someone recovering their mental health, a consistent approach can be an essential part of the care they receive.

A third point is that lack of clarity affects individual and staff group confidence in taking on new ideas and hence their capacity to change. There are wider issues here which relate to the general openness of an establishment which we will discuss when looking in more detail at the factors which influence the implementation of change.

Staff are Vulnerable to Criticism

We were made aware of how vulnerable staff can be to the possibility of criticism. There was generally a high level of anxiety about being criticised or failing on the job. This was, not surprisingly, most marked in child care establishments but all staff had a keen sense of their responsibility of care.

The consequences of such anxiety seemed to be a defensive adherence to whatever guidelines or routines were in place or a kind of abdication of responsibility. This kind of anxiety was demonstrated by, for example, the worker who was fearful that being involved in a training project would result in her having to take more responsibility.

Staff involved in IQA trials were anxious about the kind of issues that residents might raise but they were more concerned, on the whole, about the way that senior management might react. The fear of getting things wrong, the level of anxiety about 'them'—the managers who were external to the home—was a common and pervasive theme. It seemed that, for many, it was not safe to think flexibly about, or even listen to, what residents might be saying because this might conflict with the established way of doing things. Staff in this kind of establishment were not free to relate or to respond to residents in an easy and open way.

Again, the reasons why such feelings should be so marked need more research but we could not fail to notice a general caution and unwillingness on the part of unit managers to challenge senior management and on the part of care workers to speak up within the homes.

Staff Can be Unaware of or Undervalue the Skills and Knowledge That They Have

We noted a tendency for staff, as individuals and as teams, either to be unaware of or to undervalue the knowledge and skills that they have built up. There is a reservoir of experience, knowledge and skills in most establishments that can be tapped by giving staff opportunities to reflect on and share ideas about their work.

Most of the training projects showed how staff responded to the opportunity to reflect on their work with enthusiasm. They not only learnt from each other in the process but were also able to understand more about the home as a whole and value their part in its work. Although there was some scepticism about training in general and in-house, home-spun programmes in particular, the benefits of learning from and with colleagues surprised many. We noted the increase in commitment and confidence that comes from staff who are able to identify with and work as a team.

One of the implications to arise from CHI projects, is that some aspects of meeting residents' needs imply new roles for staff and, therefore, new skills and knowledge. For example, some Window in Homes work pointed to the need for outreach work with staff involved in building relationships and negotiating contacts with people and agencies outside the home. In training projects staff identified their need to know more about such aspects as bereavement counselling, advocacy, understanding mental health—work which would take them beyond the role of physical caring.

One of the findings of the CHI was, then, a strange parallel between the isolation of residents and that of staff. Just as residents can be cut off from important aspects of their lives, so staff can be divorced from exercising their own judgement about what makes people feel secure and fulfilled. The fear that accompanies feelings of isolation makes it all the harder for people—staff and residents—to speak up, even when there are obvious difficulties or damaging practices going on in the name of care.

Staff Need Help in Dealing with the Emotional Impact of the Work

An underlying issue, but one which found expression in most of the interviews and group discussions we had with care workers and, to a lesser extent, home managers, was how to manage anxiety. Irrespective of care group, staff were coping with strong feelings about their responsibilities and the stress of the work. Some of the most powerful related to fears of getting-it-wrong in the eyes of senior managers. But the emotional impact of the work came primarily from their concern for residents and their wellbeing. It was, perhaps, significant that few staff could talk in any detail about their feelings when a resident died or moved away. The atmosphere in one home, for example, was charged with sadness and upset on one visit we made but no-one could speak about the reason why. It was clear that the sudden death of an elderly resident had shocked everyone but had not brought people together. Staff kept quiet—perhaps as a way of avoiding the sadness and loss.

Staff status and morale are closely related to feeling effective, involved and valued as workers. Opportunities created through the projects for staff to come together and reflect on practice and, as important, their own experience and feelings, brought significant shifts in confidence. A key contribution of the CHI has been to demonstrate how such opportunities can help to address anxieties and problems generated by the work.

Chapter 8

QUALITY OF LIFE, CHANGE AND PARTICIPATION IN RESIDENTIAL ESTABLISHMENTS

We turn now to some general questions about promoting the quality of residents' lives and initiating the kind of changes in residential establishments and their management that may be necessary in order to do so. Do the findings of CHI provide new perspectives or prompt different thinking about well-being and quality of life? Are there general lessons to be drawn from the Initiative about what helps to ensure that people in residential care enjoy the lifestyle they prefer? What can be learnt from the different models and approaches used by the research teams to implement and manage change? The chapter explores the role of residential establishments in providing an enabling environment and concludes with the formulation of a user-led approach to service development and evaluation.

Quality of Life in Residential Establishments

Quality of life in residential care homes was the theme which permeated all the work of the Initiative but no one definition was established between the researchers, the homes and agencies which participated or ourselves as evaluators. Throughout the presentation of the work, so far, we have referred to a resident's lifestyle, to the experience of the resident, to their expectations and aspirations rather than attempt a definition of quality of life—a notion that encapsulates something that is very personal while being part of the rhetoric of public service provision.

However, in the light of the findings of the CHI as a whole, we now examine the notion of quality of life in residential care in more detail: what is meant by quality of life? can it be defined? can it be measured? what is the relationship between the quality of service provided and the quality of life experienced by the resident?

What is Meant by Quality of Life?

In thinking about quality of life we have found it helpful to make distinctions between service inputs and outputs on the one hand and outcomes for residents on the other.

Inputs are the policies, structures, activities, procedures and resources that go into providing a service. These include aspects that impinge directly on service delivery like the care practice of the staff, admission procedures, material resources, daily routines. It also includes indirect aspects: arrangements that help to support the staff—like training and supervision; systems that help to ensure that standards are set and maintained—like service reviews and monitoring. Statements about the aims and purposes of the establishment and its working philosophy are also inputs—they help to inform others about what is being provided and how. All these can be specified and checked for their relevance and effectiveness in providing the service.

Outputs are the actual accommodation and care services provided. These include both the visible, concrete aspects—like the resident's room, the meals provided, the arrangements for making complaints and the less tangible—like the climate of the place, the tenor of the relationships between staff and residents. The more concrete, the easier it is to find objective measures of service output that can be universally agreed: either there is or is not a system for making complaints, either the room has the amenities advertised or it does not. The more atmospheric aspects, however, require subjective measures and assessments will vary according to preference and perception.

Outcomes are the impacts or results of the services for the people who use them or who are affected by them in some way. Here the key sources of evaluative comment are found outside the agency and beyond those who work to provide the service. Although the people of primary importance are those for whom the service is intended, they are not the only source of feedback. Here we make some further distinctions between:

- those who directly use the service—the residents;

- those who have an obvious interest—like the relatives of residents;

- those with a less obvious interest but who can, nevertheless, be much affected by the way a service is run—like the traders who supply a care home, like neighbours and others in the locality;

- those who work in the service—like the managers, care workers and administrative staff.

A service will have an impact on all these groups of people irrespective of the intended beneficiaries. Making these distinctions enables us to separate:

- the service (inputs and outputs) *from* its effects (outcomes);

- the activities and resources involved in providing a service *from* the experience of using or receiving it; and

- the viewpoints of service providers *from* service users and other interested parties.

Quality of service

Residential care providers draw on information and ideas—from professionals, other providers and from residents themselves—about what users want and what will meet their requirements. They define the purposes and objectives of the service and the people for whom it is provided. Specifications and targets determine the design, scope, form and level of service. The extent to which a provider achieves these objectives and targets can be measured against the definitions and specifications that have been set. The quality of a service relates to its level of achievement in providing the intended output.

Quality of life

For users there are two crucial and subtly different questions to ask of any service:

- does it deliver what it promises?

- does it meet the need(s) for which it was chosen?

The first confines appraisal to the service's own frame of reference: did the service as experienced (outcome) match its intentions? Did the user get what they were led to expect? There are underlying issues here about how far a potential user is able to make a decision and form expectations of a service based on accurate and relevant information.

The second question concerns the interests of the user and their individual frame of reference. Here the relevance and standard of service is considered in relation to their particular set of needs.

In thinking about quality of life, in the context of residential services, we are essentially concerned with outcomes for the people who live in establishments. There are a number of separate issues here.

Quality of life is about the whole of someone's living experience. This includes memories of the past as well as current realities. It includes aspirations and hopes for the future as well fears or uncertainties about what is happening now. It is about feeling confident that there are people who love and care about you and about fearing rejection and isolation. The earlier discussion about social integration needs helps to highlight the importance of the inner world of thoughts and feelings alongside the activities and relationships that are more easily perceived by others. These are aspects of living experience that are not—and cannot be—totally shaped or defined by the setting or present circumstances in which someone lives.

It follows, then, that there can be no universal definition of what constitutes quality of life. It is an essentially subjective notion and one that can only be defined in idiosyncratic terms. It is the individual who knows if their experience of life is, on the whole, satisfying or incomplete, although others will see that same life in a wider or a narrower context and make judgements according to their experience and values. Others' perceptions might be helpful, challenging, supportive or they might be inaccurate, biased, irrelevant: only the individual concerned can tell. As well as being highly individual, ideas about well-being and life style also change. Preferences, needs, expectations and aspirations are volatile—they change in the light of experience and are subject to new meanings and priorities.

If we accept that there is no ideal and that notions of quality of life are essentially individual, subjective, idiosyncratic and volatile then it follows that it is not possible either to define or measure the quality of life provided or experienced within a particular establishment in any collective way. The same home may be experienced as highly satisfactory and as oppressive by different residents. Universal rights and freedoms can be understood and, to some extent, provided for on a collective basis—for example, along the lines of the principles set out in *Homes are for Living In* (DOH/SSI, 1989a). These cannot encompass all that is necessary to ensure a satisfactory life for the individual but how they are translated into day-by-day living arrangements, future plans and opportunities will either help or hinder the realisation of individual aspirations.

All this does not throw out the usefulness of the concept. In a paradoxical way it endorses the importance of paying attention to quality of life and the conditions which promote fulfilment.

The Residential Care Home as an Enabling Environment

The experience of the CHI projects suggests that the preferred lifestyle of residents might best be promoted by thinking of the establishment as an environment—a kind of base camp—within which or from which, the individual can utilise or create opportunities to grow and change, meet challenges or rest from them.

In providing services and accommodation a care establishment cannot deliver quality of life as such but it can play a part in providing the conditions and creating the opportunities by which an individual can realise the lifestyle of their choice.

A key task of the establishment is, then, to identify the conditions and opportunities which enable growth and fulfilment. Some may be appropriately found within the boundaries of the home: others may be found through community links, through social networks, in association with outside agencies or friends or political parties or a religious community or a sports club.

The point is to establish the kind of base from which these opportunities can be developed and to maintain an open and receptive approach to the changing needs and aspirations of individual residents.

The notion of a facilitating or enabling environment is taken from Winnicott (see Davis and Wallbridge, 1983). In his terms we live in a kind of paradox where, for fulfilment, each individual needs to be free to express the self and realise their own personality and, at the same time, to feel held and safe. Bowlby's idea of a safe base is similar (Bowlby, 1973). He suggests that the capacity to explore and grow, to reach out and develop, can be done most successfully when the individual (an adult just as much as a child) feels that they have a safe place or a reliable and accepting person to retreat to if things go wrong.

In terms of residential care, an enabling environment is a living situation which allows the expression of individual rights and freedoms and encourages personal fulfilment. Everyone is in some way constrained from total and uninhibited expression of their wishes: those who live in a collective or group-based situation may be more restricted than others.

Fulfilment assumes capacity for growth, adaptation, change: there is a dynamic, interactive relationship between people and their environment. There are however difficulties which flow from change: uncertainties, the need to adapt, the impact on and reactions of others. Change can be unsettling and even frightening.

A secure base on the other hand is, in some measure at least, typified by continuity. Safeness comes from the reliability, predictability, unchanging-ness of a known person or situation. The less welcome aspect of safeness is that it may come to represent a fixed, limiting, confining state which is also difficult to challenge. What might happen if you upset the continuity? the unchangingness? What are the risks?

The Wagner review highlighted both change and continuity as key elements in providing quality of life. One of the Post Wagner Development Group (WDG) working groups, for example, looked at the the complex issue of security of tenure for people entering a residential establishment (see NISW/HMSO, 1993). Equally, the possibilities of being able to review, make choices and change were at the heart of many of the recommenda-tions of the original review and subsequent commentaries from the WDG.

Putting these ideas together with the ideas about the experience of residents which we discussed in the last chapter suggests that an enabling environment is likely to be one which tackles both continuity and change and recognises the different interests involved and the provision of service. Table 8.1 sets out the main features of an enabling establishment.

Table 8.1—The Residential Care Home as an Enabling Environment

An enabling establishment is one in which:

• it is accepted that group-based residential living cannot replicate living in one's own home: there are essential differences in collective provision. Some of these have positive potential for growth, for the realisation of reciprocal relationships, for the self-realisation of the individual: some have negative effects requiring compromise or the subjugation of individual goals;

• people—staff and residents—recognise and value differences and seek to meet individual preferences;

• conflicts of interest are recognised as an intrinsic element of collective living and working and these are made explicit and available for debate;

• quality of life is understood in individual terms;

• continuity and reliability are respected;

• change is seen as a necessary and intrinsic part of everyday living: to accommodate new members, to meet changing demands, to adapt to the different stages in the life cycle of its members, to react to fresh ideas from inside and from outside;

• development and setting standards of good practice have no end point: a care home cannot 'get it right' once and for all;

• it is acknowledged that ability to meet and adapt appropriately to change requires an open culture—one in which staff and residents are open and undefensive about new ideas and perceptions;

• it is recognised that the living base, its facilities and services represent only a part of the individual's living experience: an establishment cannot assume responsibility for providing a total environment;

• a sense of security comes from clarity about the terms on which the accommodation and services are available. Even where security of tenure cannot be guaranteed people have a right to know where they stand and the conditions of residence;

• community resources and opportunities are fully available to residents;

• it is assumed that people can speak for themselves or can be enabled to do so with appropriate support;

• residents and staff participate in reviews and decision making about how the home is run;

• staff are well trained and supported and valued for their contribution to review and development.

Questions of balance

These features suggest that the enabling residential establishment has two key tasks:

- maintaining a balance between continuity and change;

- establishing ways of balancing the different interests represented in a collective living and working situation.

There are a number of balances to be considered: between individuals and a collective, between residents and staff, between internal and external interests. The different levels of interest affect each other and each can alter the relative equilibrium of the establishment towards change or towards greater stability. This goes some way to demonstrating the complexity of the tasks and why apparently minor shifts or changes can have a significant impact. Implicit in feedback from project workers and participants was that it does not help if such complexities are denied or over-simplified.

The experience of the projects suggests that there are two important aspects of tackling these tasks: that difficulties are recognised rather than denied and that those with a primary stake in the home—residents, relatives, care staff and managers—are involved in review and decision making wherever possible.

Measuring Quality of Life
These ideas provide ways of checking how quality of life issues are tackled by establishments even if individual satisfaction cannot easily be measured or even directly attributed to the situation in the home.

Three questions provide the basis of an assessment of quality of lifestyle and opportunities for fulfilment:

- does the establishment provide an enabling environment for the individual as well as the resident group?

- does the establishment seek to recognise and mediate appropriately between different interests?

- are there opportunities for individual as well as collective feedback and commentary?

Change and Innovation in Residential Services

Much of what we have presented so far is about change: in care practice, in the way needs are defined and met, in management approaches, in attitudes to and understanding of the care task, in the way services are provided. The work of the CHI projects showed how, in many homes, the involvement of frontline staff and residents in reviewing current practice, revealed the need for change: new perspectives, priorities and opportunities for development were recognised.

The main strand of our discussion is to consider how far innovation at the grassroots can be effective in meeting quality objectives. Again the key themes which we explore concern the resident: in what ways are care establishments able—and enabled—to ensure that service developments are led by user interests?

Initiating Change from the Grassroots

What do the CHI projects tell us about change from the grassroots? How feasible is it for local managers and individual care homes to take the initiative both in defining need for change and taking action? How successful are local developments in ensuring that residents' interests are primary?

Important questions about change and development relate to:

- initiating change from the grassroots

- how the agenda for change is set and by whom

- mediating between interests

- initiation and implementation

- how changes are sustained.

Initiating change

There was, generally, a high level of enthusiasm for tackling the projects. Care home managers and proprietors were interested in developing something new, even at a time of upheaval, and most particularly valued the opportunity to take some initiative. The CHI projects provided the stimulus for change but, in many cases, the motivation for change was already there. This stemmed from the changes taking place in community care but there were also managers who were focusing on the needs of residents. Many were uncertain how to proceed or even if they had the authority to do so.

There was a positive response to the idea that care homes could and should be taking the initiative in defining and making changes to meet local needs and demands. There was enthusiasm from frontline staff for taking some control of how the home developed, for setting priorities and taking action. A grassroots approach appealed to peoples' knowledge of 'their' residents, homes and locale.

A key question to be asked is whether some form of outside stimulus is necessary to prompt change. The more settled the home the less likely it is, perhaps, to recognise the need for development. Regular in-house review is significant here: IQA projects demonstrated how the views of residents often surprised staff. In this way the essential stimuli for change can come from within as well as from outside.

There was, then, widespread affirmation for initiating change at the level of the care home but also a recognition that this required some form of validation either from within the agency or from outside. There are underlying issues of authority, leadership and confidence here which we will take up later. But the projects confirmed that the individual home could take the initiative and with positive results.

Setting the agenda

Most of the projects used some form of audit to look at current practice and consider what action might need to be taken. The assumption was that frontline managers could initiate a process of internal review that would guide action for improving the service. In this way the agenda for change was based on the views and experience of local managers and staff and, in many cases, residents as well. Frontline workers were not only involved but also had a direct understanding of what action might be desirable and a sense of ownership and commitment to the changes planned. As a result, the projects were seen as highly relevant and, at least to some extent, under the control of the people who knew most about the work. It was evident that managers appreciated the flexibility of devising and reflecting on their own strategies for change and that staff were better able to see the connection between new approaches and the objectives being pursued. Even where staff were not closely involved in review and planning there was an acceptance that the plans were being developed by accessible and known colleagues. The possibilities of staff dissociating themselves from, or undermining, changes by attributing them to distant managers with unknown motives were reduced.

In a number of projects the review provided opportunities for residents to be involved. This was most clearly achieved in the IQA work but was a point for discussion in many homes. What the IQA reviews suggest is that some structured opportunity may well be required to ensure that residents can give their views. Generally, there was little to suggest that the potential of resident committees or meetings to contribute to overall review and planning was being explored.

Mediating and balancing interests

The issue then is how different perceptions and priorities can be accommodated or balanced. Again, the IQA experience points to the value of including rather than excluding those who have an interest in the way the home is run and developed. The recognition of relatives and carers as well as residents and staff helps to ensure change is not defined is an over-simple way that fails to take account of potentially conflicting demands, ideas or priorities.

The difficulties of defining and balancing the direction and priorities for change may be off-set by the understanding (even if in dissent) and commitment that results when people are included and involved.

It is a management task to make decisions about the running of the homes but nearly all projects involved a series of meetings to discuss progress, to revise objectives and time scales and to provide feedback to staff and to residents. Many homes used resident meetings in this way.

Initiating and pursuing change

Deciding on how to pursue changes was usually the most complicated part of the projects. In considering the training work we noted that a crucial stage was designing the programme to implement the training plan and that it was here that establishments needed most help. The issues were to clarify what the home could initiate without reference to or help from the wider organisation and not to take on problems that belonged elsewhere.

One of the most important aspects to emerge was that people appreciated the control they had over the time scale and pace of change. People were aware of the dangers of losing focus and impetus over time but these were offset by the value of the work. Indeed, a number of homes continued doggedly despite delays and difficulties: their commitment stemmed from their conviction that what they were doing was worthwhile.

Sustaining change

Although the CHI consultants were important in initiating the projects, sustaining the work was in the hands of local managers and staff. The greater the sense of purpose that built up around the work, the more likely it was that people wanted to continue.

The projects were seen as particularly worthwhile where residents were involved or benefited significantly from the work.

Where the projects involved other agencies or helped to establish networks of interest there were external supports as well as internal reasons for continuing the work.

What Helps Openness to Change and the Capacity to Respond?

These points, together with earlier discussion, begin to identify some of the features of care provision, practice and management that help a residential establishment to be open to change.

Clarity about the philosophy and purposes of the home

We noted earlier that in many homes staff did not have a confident understanding of the purposes of the establishment. People could quote the broad aims but with little deeper appreciation of what this meant in practical terms: there was no shared philosophy to help them think about everyday tasks and how to work with each other. In some cases, the difficulties resulting from this had led to serious rifts in staff teams.

It is not only researchers who notice such difficulties: residents are quickly aware of tensions in a staff group: the more their well-being depends on the staff the more frightening staff disagreements can be. Residents told us, poignantly, about how they had to adapt according to 'who was on'.

Equally, there was evidence from across the projects that the clearer staff were about the tasks they were undertaking and the greater their sense of working together, the more confident they were in their relationships with residents: staff at all levels were more flexible, less afraid of failure and more likely to listen to residents' ideas and views. This confidence seemed also to result in people feeling more prepared to take responsibility rather than avoid a problem, push it further up the organisation or onto someone else.

But although ensuring clarity about the work is a responsibility of local managers, this has to be supported by clarity in the organisation as a whole. In a Window in Homes project, for example, staff felt unable to proceed with plans to help their residents with learning disabilities to get out and about more until the agency had worked out a policy on risk taking. The staff needed to know that senior managers understood the implications of promoting greater independence for residents and were asking the agency to take responsibility.

Openness to change and receptivity to new ideas flow, then, from opportunities to reflect with and to build trust in colleagues and develop clarity about the need for development. Fears of 'getting it wrong' can easily lead to defensive and rigid—unchanging—practice.

Home as a whole
A common feature in the way Programmes approached their work was in thinking about establishments as whole units. The use of an audit or review was a way of emphasising the importance of this—whether the aim was to produce a training plan, to understand more about the home's links with the community or was undertaken as part of an overall IQA review. One of the results was that managers and staff had the opportunity to consider their work in the round. This reflection had the effect, in nearly all cases, of raising awareness of the home as whole—a place with a purpose and of great importance to the people who live and work there. There were numbers of junior staff who commented on how much they did not know about how their home was run: feeling part of a home that has a clear identity and which is valued helped to create a climate in which staff themselves felt valued.

There were indications that homes which had a strong sense of identity and purpose were those which were more outward looking and least isolated.

Leadership and the culture of the home
In nearly all the homes we visited, it appeared that the head of the home was most influential in determining the climate and culture of the establishment.

Staff and residents invariably explained to us how a home had changed when a new manager came. Although they spoke of changes in physical arrangements, routines and procedures, in the main they described a significant shift in the climate and working culture: attitudes, expectations and working relationships had changed and with them the general ambience of the home.

The CHI projects did not focus directly on leadership nor on how the climate of a home is created. But it was clear that the role of the manager was crucial in setting people's expectations about how work should be done and how the home should run. Residents as well as staff looked to the head of the home to guide the way they related to other people.

A climate of openness can be strongly influenced, therefore, by the attitude and approach of the head of the establishment: the more confident they are, the more likely it is that they will be able to listen to and value the contribution of others.

Preparedness to question traditions and established ways

Another aspect of openness to change is that it implies a preparedness to question, and if necessary, give up old ways. We have referred to a number of ways in which traditional notions of care, established professional views and current patterns of service provision, each based on particular assumptions about people's need and wishes, can be a barrier to understanding and responding to users' current needs.

A key question here is to ask how new ideas enter the system. How do changing needs become apparent and how do shifts in people's expectations and aspirations become known? The work of IQA has shown how involving residents and carers can have a strong influence on the way residential services are run. User and carer organisations have always been active in providing information and campaigning for services and rights. There were indications from the PSI work that their role is being recognised by service planners and providers as a valuable source of information about needs, trends in demand and current thinking about good practice. In the future it could well be the consumers—residents and relatives in their different ways—who will ensure that rigid practices and patterns of service will be challenged and replaced by reflective management and flexible responses.

Enhancing links with community and local agencies

Window in Homes projects focused particularly on enhancing local links. Other Programmes worked with clusters of homes or agencies as a way of pooling resources or developing local networks for a particular client group. One of the lessons to emerge from the varied experience of these projects was that looking outside the home for support and for exchange of knowledge, brought many benefits.

For example, people in the field of mental health gained an understanding of other services and realised a new and valued identity as mental health workers, by joining a training network. The staff and their agencies were exposed to and learnt from the views and ideas of others in their own field of provision: many said they felt better able to understand their residents as a result. There were benefits, too, in reducing the sense of isolation that affects so many care homes as managers and staff met workers from other establishments.

Working with outsiders was a feature of the IQA review and here too people referred to the stimulation of fresh ideas. As well as individuals, there is potential here for local user and consumer organisations to take a role in representing the interests of different care groups, carers and relatives to service providers.

An underlying question relates to how far managers feel it is a legitimate use of their time to make external links of this sort. It is likely that all establishments will become more outward looking in order to maintain their reputation, professional networks, community care arrangements and to increase consumer awareness and participation.

Support from the agency and freedom to act

Homes in large organisations required the support and backing of management and the wider agency. If this was not clear, then local innovation could be difficult to justify in the first place or hard to sustain.

Significant evidence for the lack of appropriate management, absence or ambiguity of support, inconsistency of expectations and lack of understanding of the complexities of the residential task came from nearly all the project consultants we met. This emerged as an underlying motivation for involvement in CHI work: managers saw a legitimate way of demonstrating to senior management or management committees how their home could develop given the support and scope to do so. Working with a CHI agency was attractive since it gave the work authority and some extra resources.

Some care home managers were faced with the anomaly of being unable to act without higher authority on relatively minor issues while, at the same time, being unsupported in dealing with significant problems. Managers also spoke of frustration when senior managers were not committed or experienced enough to understand the work of residential care and, therefore, the nature of particular difficulties they faced. There were instances where it was clear that a home was seen by senior management as one of a cluster for which blanket decisions and arrangements could be made, rather than an establishment in its own locale, with its own set of relationships and specific demands to be met.

In a significant number of cases managers were uncertain about how far, in normal circumstances, they would be allowed by their agency (or the proprietor) to try something new or take active steps to develop the work of their home. This lack of clarity led to the kind of situation where managers and staff either did not have the confidence to innovate, or were apathetic or did not feel such things were their responsibility.

In looking at the work of Window in Homes we discussed the need for more outreach on the part of home staff and, in some cases, an active role in working with outside agencies. This implies a degree of local autonomy to act and to respond to local opportunities and situations as they arise either for the home as a whole or to support the individual resident.

Lack of clarity about the degree of discretion that could be exercised by the head of a home or poor support from line managers contributed to the difficulties of a considerable number of homes. Nearly all the managers in our case studies, for example, referred to ambiguities in their role, to lack of consistency in management approaches and expectations and some also thought that their line and senior mangers had little understanding of residential services. For some this amounted to a serious mismatch between their ideas about how to do the job and those of senior managers. If managers are not sure of their role and authority it becomes impossible for them to help a staff team to develop a coherent or consistent approach to the work.

The work of CHI Programmes did not address organisational and management issues directly. The contribution that the approaches make is in highlighting the impact, at local level, of particular policies and resource decisions made elsewhere in the organisation. Innovation at, and feedback from, grassroots is likely to entail a critique of current policies and priorities. There were some indications from IQA projects that the more service users are involved in review and are able to voice opinions, the more influence grassroots experience is likely to have within the providing agency. However, the structures to enable this to happen and the kind of cultural shift needed to ensure messages are understood and taken up are hardly in place at the current time.

Towards User-led Service Development and Evaluation

The concern throughout the work and our evaluation has been to promote quality in ways that serve the interests of the resident.

The approaches explored by the CHI projects embrace a number of features which, put together, begin to offer an approach to service appraisal and development which is user-led. Although we refer to residents, the issues relate to the wider community care framework and have relevance for other forms of service and other settings.

The model is based on three ideas each linked to residents' values and interests.

• First, there is no end point to residential service development. An establishment cannot reach a situation where a quality service has been established. Services able to meet individual needs and aspirations are responsive and flexible: they cannot be static and unchanging.

• Second, is the notion that quality is not an achievement but a process of development guided by the values and objectives of those who use the service. To be effective, the processes and practices entailed in pursuing quality must be interactive and negotiative rather than pre-scriptive, and involve those with a stake in the outcomes of the service. Different interests are recognised and balanced but those of the resident are primary.

• Linking these notions is the third. Residents as individuals and as members of a group have rights and responsibilities to participate in the processes by which service objectives and standards are set, imple-mented and evaluated.

Much of current policy development draws on a consumer model for service provision. The NHS and Community Care Act 1990, for example, makes connections between consumer mechanisms like contracting and purchasing of services—which are based on a market philosophy—and choice and quality of services. In its ideal form, this assumes an exchange of goods or services where there is open and rational choice, with neutral and equal bargaining points and open access to information and decision making networks. It is already clear that services are not equivalent to goods in a market place and purchasers of services are agencies or professionals rather than the direct users. Arguably, even residents who are direct purchasers of care (such as elderly people paying for a place in a private home) are not in this situation. In residential care we are also dealing with people's homes, so that quality is a matter of quality of users' lives. The security of people living in residential care is a key issue here.

What is implied by the CHI experience is different in nature from a consumer model of service provision, even though the policy climate of consumerism may support it. The principle is, rather, one of residents' rights and responsibilities to participate in the decisions and practices which affect their lives, to make choices within the possibilities available and to argue for extending these possibilities. This follows the view that only individuals can define the quality of their own lives: the externally defined quality of a good or service cannot determine or guarantee the experience of the service user.

Are there alternative principles to that of consumerism which can underpin a user model of service provision?

One important principle is that of citizenship. Although rarely defined, this is a concept with legal, social and moral aspects which encompasses basic rights of welfare and representation. Unlike the consumer concept, it focuses more on communal responsibility for quality of service provision and for opportunities for people to participate in community life. Citizen-ship implies both rights and responsibilities for participation in society and in political processes at all levels. People who live in institutional settings have often been denied such rights, a denial which stems from seeing those who need care or support as somehow less than a person, or an adult, with full citizenship rights.

Reciprocity is also an important principle to consider here. Living in residential care is generally associated with notions of dependency, which are linked to our ideas about care. Reciprocity, on the other hand, suggests giving as well as receiving. It implies greater equality and the possibility of contribution through, for example, becoming more involved in everyday running of an establishment or in outside activities. Reciprocity, like citizenship, is an important aspect of having recognised social roles. More than this, it counters assumptions about total dependency which encourage service providers to view people as categories defined by their care needs.

Towards User Participation

Voice

There is a fundamental distinction between service providers adopting a *user orientation* and direct *user participation* in service review and development. Consultation, for example, means asking for people's views but participation implies, in addition, their direct involvement in decision making and action.

There is considerable value, as we saw in the NISW projects, in providers and practitioners developing a greater sensitivity to users' needs and thinking about services in relation to user interests. There were indications from projects that staff were able to re-appraise long held views and take on new perceptions if the opportunities to do so were led or validated by people they respected. Such shifts in attitudes and assumptions led to greater awareness of residents' needs and wishes and were effective in moving homes towards user involvement.

However, taking a user orientation, on the evidence of the projects and other research findings (e.g. Le Touze and Pahl, 1990) is unlikely to be enough on its own. The views of providers and users can differ widely. Providers' ideas can easily become out of date, patronising or stereotyped. We frequently heard staff say 'we know what our residents want/like/need' even where there were no opportunities for discussion with or feedback from residents.

Choice

Involving users requires individual and collective means of promoting choice. Individual choices are made within a framework bound by the collective residential situation—limits may be imposed by institutional requirements such as cost, scale, essential management functions, sharing of home space with others including paid carers. They may also be imposed by collective considerations—individual choices do sometimes conflict so that compromise and accommodation is necessary. The present situation is that choice is often limited by unnecessary organisational routines and patterns. Areas which the CHI Programmes might have explored further are the role of residents' groups and the potential of individual and collective advocacy in enabling residents to speak out. The IQA system of review encapsulates a way of balancing interests which is geared, as far as possible, towards residents' interests, rather than simply governed by organisational considerations.

Participation

Participation needs to progress from individual to collective issues. Starting with the individual helps to ensure their wishes and feelings are heard. More collective work recognises the shared setting of services but also the differences of interest between groups with differing power and influence. Likewise, there are different levels of choice and involvement possible for current and prospective users of residential care:

The first level includes:-
    assessment for residential (or other) services;
    choice of a residential care home;
    admission to a residential care home.

The second level is about everyday choices for the individual and includes:-
    personal care;
    personal lifestyle and cultural preferences;
    management of everyday life, routines etc.;
    choice, initiation and location of activities.

The third level is about participation and choice affecting the way the service is run and includes:-
    patterns of staffing and staff selection;
    decision making within services;
    how changes are planned;
    use of space and time;
    relationships with other users and staff;
    who to share a home with;
    a role in quality assurance and review.

Moving towards the third level requires structures for collective and continuing representation and participation. The user voice in a particular service, therefore, will be facilitated by positive staff support, but also require connection with agency decision-making processes.

Effective communication at all levels is based on people having sufficient knowledge of their rights, about how to express preferences, of the services available and alternative possibilities. Lack of information can prevent people from making choices and disable participation.

Enabling user participation

Although, increasingly, services are canvassing user views and taking active steps to obtain feedback, these have tended to take the form of surveys carried out at a particular time for particular agency purposes: the information is valuable but limited. There is a considerable difference between a one-off survey of this sort and involving users in dialogue and feedback as an integral, everyday part of the culture and management of the home (Youll and Perring, 1991). Participation requires *established and regular*, as well as informal or occasional, opportunities for involvement.

The difficulty which many residents experience in saying what needs to change has highlighted the *need for information*. To make choices effective and to prevent the development of low expectations amongst those receiving care, people require to up-to-date knowledge. Often, service users are unaware of alternatives and uncomfortable about appearing to moan, particularly when staff 'work so hard' . The user's power to comment, or to complain, is further limited by the restricted rights and security of those in residential care and by their very dependence on the care which is available.

Service development that is led by user concerns does, then, require their direct involvement and on a regular integrated basis. Some of the practicalities of this and the constraints to achieving effective participation have been evident though our discussion of the Initiative.

A user-led approach is one in which it is recognised that there are *differences of power and interest* between groups with a stake in the service and that service users have generally been the least powerful and the least heard. The experience of IQA suggests that structures and procedures are required if opportunities for residents to speak up are to be systematic and sustained.

User participation requires *legitimation* as well as opportunities to speak out. The user voice within an establishment may well be more effective where it is recognised—by staff and residents—that there is a strong external voice expressing the interests of the user group. In Chapter 2 we noted that the strength and degree of development of user organis-ations, and the extent to which they have captured public attention and awareness, varies across care groups. It remains the case, for example, that elders in residential establishments have little or no organised voice although there are a numerous voluntary agencies representing the interests of elderly people generally. In contrast, children in care are successfully asserting their right to be heard and organisations like NAYPIC are regularly consulted on policy and practice issues. User and advocacy organisations can play a direct role in publicising their views and facilitat-ing others to do so at more local levels. They also have a more indirect impact in fostering an ethos where service providers acknowledge the value of user consultation and participation. The voice and visibility of such groups could encourage residents to form their own groups and to give their individual views.

User participation, rather than simple consultation or developing a user orientation, requires a greater degree of organisational change and has far reaching implications for *the way services are planned and managed*. It should allow the principles of consultation and choice to become aspects of everyday life.

It involves significant *shifts in attitude* as well as more formal arrangements. There is an interesting question, which the CHI projects were not able to answer, about where to begin. Jones, writing about women in the police comments:

'It is much easier to initiate change in the social structure or in the technical components than it is at the cultural level. In short, attitudes die hard.'

(Jones, 1986).

Table 8.2—Conditions and Arrangements for User Participation

A Values:
- individual rights
- recognition of multiple interests
- participation in the processes of service review and development
- power sharing

B Culture:
- open and responsive
- acceptance of change
- balance between continuity and change
- acceptance of difference
- integration rather than segregation
- collaborative and negotiative relationships
- open exchange of information and knowledge

C Organisation:
- opportunities for communication between interest groups
- structures for direct participation
- resources for user participation
- balancing collective and individual demands
- lateral rather than hierarchical connections
- local autonomy
- clear and accessible complaints procedures

D Policy environment:
- consumer rights and advocacy
- tenancy and citizenship rights
- individual needs-led assessment
- service contract specifications include arrangements for user participation.

These points echo some of the conclusions drawn by Parsloe and Stevenson from their recent study of the empowerment of users and carers. (Parsloe and Stevenson, 1993). They emphasised the need to acknowledge the complexity of the issues relating to ensuring that service users have a voice. In particular they pointed out that changes were required throughout an organisation—not just frontline staff—if greater user participation was to be achieved and sustained.

A user-led approach does not imply that external systems of quality control are not necessary. It acknowledges that these are needed to establish norms including the basic requirements of acceptable practice. Within such frameworks participative approaches to promoting quality may have a better chance of being effective, and being sustained. The expectations of users are strongly influenced by their experiences and so may be very low in some situations but we have seen how being involved, in itself, can begin to alter those expectations.

Putting these observations together we arrive at a list of the kind of conditions and arrangements that are needed to provide service users with the opportunity to participate in and influence service development. They rest on three key elements: consultation, knowledge and rights and these are set out in Table 8.2.

The work of the Programmes did not alter the boundaries of choice but has demonstrated ways in which possibilities for greater voice and choice may be opened out. The positive developments we have seen imply certain forms of organisation and activity. The principle of participation can be applied throughout the service system—from styles of management and training to structures for user involvement and information exchange. At all levels, and whatever the task, the keys are clarity of principles and purpose and sharing of power so that responsibility, too, may be shared. There is a connection between an enabling environment for those living in residential care and an enabling environment for those who provide care.

Chapter 9

DEVELOPMENTAL ISSUES AND IMPLICATIONS FOR RESIDENTIAL SERVICE PROVIDERS AND USERS

The aims of the Initiative were to explore how the recommendations of the Wagner review might be implemented and to demonstrate how the quality of life of people living in residential establishments might be assured. In previous chapters we discussed the main achievements and some of the limitations of the research and presented an overview of the findings of the Initiative as a whole. We focused on the experience of residents and looked at quality from their point of view. We considered how residential services might develop in order to ensure that residents' needs and aspirations are understood and responded to. In this final chapter we identify some of the developmental issues highlighted by the CHI and consider their implications for those who use, shape and provide services.

Developmental Trends and Issues

The CHI Programmes developed ideas and approaches to practice designed to promote the interests of residents across the care groups. In doing so, the researchers worked closely with people in the front line of service in order to develop ideas and practice: the issues which emerged in the course of the work can be summarised as they relate to different levels and interests.

- Ensuring quality of service is strongly related to how the preferred lifestyle of residents is defined and understood. The work of the Programmes pointed to the need for a more individualised approach to meeting social and care needs.

- Quality of life is strongly linked to personal relationships, opportunities for growth and self-fulfilment. The social and emotional isolation of people living in establishments is not being fully recognised or responded to.

- The categorisation of people according to their age or ability is being challenged by residents and by user and other organisations which represent their interests. The user movement generally and, increasingly, the views expressed by residents themselves and through their advocates, are pushing service development further in the direction of individual planning and provision.

• There is a trend away from using long established care group categories which define people and determine their eligibility for service. We found no evidence that users wanted to dismantle the services that have traditionally served people with particular needs: rather that these should be organised so that they can be more flexible and not necessarily provided in a particular (eg residential) setting.

• There is a trend away from providing total care within the home towards making full use of ordinary facilities and opportunities available in the locality.

• It follows that residential establishments will become more open and flexible in the way they offer and provide accommodation, care and other services.

• The importance of knowing about services, of access to and open exchange of information is becoming widely appreciated. It will take a long time before residents, potential residents or their relatives are 'informed consumers' (Allen et al 1992) able to question, choose between available alternatives and comment fully on the services they receive. We noted, however, that younger adults in residential establishments tend to be more questioning and demanding than older people.

• Care establishments are becoming more aware of what is happening locally. The trend is towards ensuring that the home's services are known about and that it has a good reputation in the area. Demonstrating quality to outsiders—whether direct purchasers or fundholders—is of increasing importance to those who run homes across the sectors.

• As care establishments become more integrated with other services and networks in the local community, the development of residential services will be more strongly influenced by and connected with local professional, user, provider and market networks and relationships.

Implications for Providers

There are a number of implications arising from these issues for those providing residential services.

Providing Residential Services
An important shift that is implied in this analysis is away from centralised decision making and management and towards greater local discretion in running residential homes.

The general view of local authority Social Service Departments and large voluntary organisations to emerge from our fieldwork is that public and independent provision is led and developed from the centre. Policies and plans are defined at the top: individual establishments are resourced and managed as part of a set of wider organisational objectives. Care homes relate to the centre through lines of management: they expect operational guidance and control from senior levels. The discretion which the care home manager can exercise is limited to the extent that decisions about the purposes of the home, working practices, staffing, budgeting, resource allocation and management are taken higher up the organisation.

The direction of much of the project work—particularly in embracing user involvement—was towards greater local connection and the discretion to pursue this. There were a number of indications from the projects that establishments were limited by being an outpost of a larger organisation rather than a unit with its own identity and autonomy. An apparent paradox was that managers were seeking greater autonomy while also complaining about lack of support. However, there is a qualitative difference between having the authority to exercise discretion and being isolated within a large organisation. The former state arises from defined and understood relationships which connect the establishment to the objectives of the agency as a whole: the latter arises from a dislocation of, or lack of clarity about, organisational relationships.

Many establishments involved in CHI projects were run by owner-proprietors. As solo operators they had freedom to work and make their own decisions at the local level but they too faced disadvantages. For example, individual homes tended to be isolated from other providers and from professional and training networks. They could lack local knowledge of policy trends, demographic changes or developments in other services. Although associations of care home managers and proprietors are widely valued, few have so far attracted the membership of a high percentage of the homes operating in their area. Individual managers and proprietors were beginning to reach out to make contact with others but many lacked resources of time and knowledge to do so effectively. Finding and using local resources and making connections often meant revising opinions—for example about the local Social Services Department—or seeing possible competitors in a new light.

In crude terms, it appeared that individual establishments and those which were part of a larger agency were recognising the benefits—if not the necessity—of stronger links with, and responsiveness to, local networks and interests. For both this meant outreach and the formation of new relationships. But both also signalled the need for a balance between responsiveness to local interests and taking account of a wider set of concerns like, for example, policy changes and requirements, national standards and expectations, social norms and professional developments.

The Meaning of Quality

The work of the Initiative points to the importance of recognising that there are many ways of viewing services and that there are multiple interests involved in the provision and outcomes of residential services. Taking the interests of residents as primary does not mean that others are not valid or to be taken into account. It does mean that there will be, in most cases, different perceptions about what constitutes quality. This leads us to suggest that residents' interests will be best served if quality of service is seen as a negotiated order which cannot be specified as a total care output or achievement. It is, rather, an agreed set of objectives, and a shared view about the means and opportunities required to pursue them.

Participation

Although consultation with users and their involvement is now widely accepted in principle, few organisations—including many of those which claim to represent user interests—have achieved much in practice. Statutory and voluntary agencies lack knowledge and experience of how to involve users, how to ensure effective consultation or how to set up structures for participation. The CHI Programme guidelines provide ideas and practice-based approaches for taking these aspects forward at the grassroots.

We suggest, however, as Parsloe and Stevenson (1993) observed, it is not only at the front line that such issues have to be addressed. It is an organisational commitment which is needed. We note in this respect the recent setting up of a users' and carers' watchdog by the Department of Health. This is a significant move at the policy level which provides a model of how different interests can contribute to debate and the formulation of policy and service development. It is a move which should stimulate service agencies to consider the various ways in which user and carer interests can be represented at different levels.

The Enabling Organisation

The CHI experience indicates some of the features that are required if an organisation is to tackle such issues. If residential establishments are to be responsive to local demands and integrated with other care services, the oganisation as a whole has to empower frontline staff. The brief points which follow are not comprehensive and they are not intended to describe an ideal type of organisation. But they move discussion to the level of organisational arrangements and responsibilities. They add up to an extension of the notion of facilitation or enablement. Just as in Chapter 8 we discussed the task of the care establishment in terms of providing an enabling environment for the resident, so the task of the organisation can be seen, in turn, as that of enabling the individual establishment to function. The more the organisation enables and gives discretion to frontline managers the more responsive the service can be to the needs of residents and can ensure their participation. What is implied is that the organisation develops in relation to grassroot experience as well as upholding certain values and mediating between the local level and wider frameworks and demands.

Features of an enabling organisation include:

• Devolvement of responsibility: decisions are made as near the ground as possible in order to involve those most directly concerned. There is an expectation that service development, establishing reputation, managing relationships with other agencies, with purchasers and potential consumers, understanding user, carer and other interests are led from the grassroots;

• The essential role of the leadership is to define the purposes and values of the organisation and to ensure that those who work within it understand and have a commitment to them;

• Recruitment for responsibility: a responsibility of the leadership is to recruit people who have the ability and can be trusted to translate these principles and values into action at the local level;

• Information exchange and a culture of openness: the purposes and policies of the organisation are clear and made public, information is provided to support outside relationships, to exchange views and knowledge and to enable participation. Within the organisation information is exchanged to ensure dialogue between different sections and to enable people to work together;

• Collaboration with outside interests: opportunities are created for debate with key outside interests including user organisations and those for relatives and families of residents. Relationships with outsiders are collaborative and negotiative;

• Receptive to grassroots: information, experience and ideas from the grassroots are valued and considered for their wider application and relevance;

• Training for responsibility and collaboration: the training culture is one which fosters collaborative—including cross-sector and multi-disciplinary—working and team development rather than individualised training and practice;

• External views and inspection: welcoming and responsive to external views both formal and informal, utilises formal inspection for developmental as well as quality control purposes;

- User participation is understood as essential in service review and development. Policies and structures enable participation, involvement in decision making and, therefore, appropriate power sharing.

Implications for Residents and User Organisations

If this analysis of trends and issues in service provision is valid then one of the main implications for those who use residential and other services is that they should expect to play an increasing role in the definition, development and evaluation of services.

The IQA system advocates that the report which is written following the review could be made available to inform outsiders—whether senior agency managers, inspectors or the general public—about the home. This is a way of giving out information about what is on offer, about the way a home is run, about how residents are involved in quality review and plans for the future. It is also one of the intentions of inspection procedures that reports should be made publicly available—for example, through local libraries. It may be some time before reports are easily accessible or widely known about as a source of information but, increasingly, these documents can be obtained.

The more that this kind of detailed information about individual homes is available, the easier it will be for user organisations, those representing user interests and individuals, to gather information about the life and work of particular establishments and draw up a profile of the nature and standards of provision in any geographical area. The possibility of more active consumer involvement is increased by such moves.

At the individual level the IQA work has shown that people from all care groups can contribute to an in-house review. This is a powerful finding—it means that there are few good reasons why anyone should be excluded from the opportunity to put their point of view. The notion of participation or power sharing may not be attractive for all residents but the potential is there. Projects showed that home managers and proprietors are concerned about reputation and that active resident involvement, far from being threatening, actually enhanced their quality image in most cases.

It seems that, for all the current limitations on resident choice and, therefore, in consumer power, there are openings for groups and individuals to articulate their views and wishes. There are certainly good reasons, on the evidence of the projects, for people to have more confidence in taking this kind of initiative.

Speaking Out

Perhaps the most significant contribution of the Initiative is in pointing up and overcoming some of the difficulties involved in ensuring that people can have a say. The hub of the work was in exploring the experience and views of people living and working in establishments. Unless they had been able to discuss their ideas and reflect on the work, there would have been few useful results. Speaking out was, then, at the heart of the research. It is at the heart of ensuring that establishments are, on the whole, good places to live and work and that they provide scope and support for growth and fulfilment whatever one's age, ability, fears or aspirations.

The indications from recent scandals were that staff and residents had asked questions, had protested but they had not been heard or taken seriously. The title of this book, 'Raising Voices', was chosen to highlight this fundamental aspect of ensuring quality: people need to be reassured that speaking out is not only a right and responsibility but that they will be heard. Care home managers and senior staff cannot afford to ignore the importance of enabling people to speak out—staff as much as residents— and taking serious note of the views and information they contribute. The person who has had an experience of being listened to is someone who is more likely to talk about their wishes or worries in future. Someone who has been silenced, or had their views dismissed once, cannot be relied on to speak out again, even against gross malpractice.

The Way Forward?

All that we have said endorses the idea that providing a quality of service and, through this, ensuring that people can pursue the lifestyle they choose, rests on understanding the nature of residential establishments. The experience of living and working in a group setting—the benefits and limitations—are common to all care groups. We saw few fundamental differences between the needs and aspirations of elders, adults with physical disabilities, abused youngsters or people with chronic mental health problems. All faced barriers and difficulties of one sort or another: each required some form of support in order to move forward. Equally,the staff we met spoke of similar hopes and concerns across the sectors and groups. What staff shared, it seemed, was a heightened sense of responsibility: there was a universal fear of the consequences of 'getting it wrong'. Residents' fears of rejection were matched by staff fears of failing to protect and care.

Opportunities for reflection, discussion or sharing activities seemed to offer a way through some of these anxieties. The essence of good practice—meeting the needs and wishes of residents—lies in discussing and reviewing what help is essential on the one hand and, on the other, discovering how little support is needed if people are confident about 'having a go' for themselves. This implies a degree of trust and cooperation between staff and residents. Imagination, flexibility and responsible reflection are to be valued rather more than prescribed practices that can be defined in manuals and packages or measured by checklists. The approaches of the CHI Programmes are based in planning and action as a result of grassroots, in-house review. They value and promote the involvement of frontline workers and, in doing, foster clarity of purpose and commitment to the work. It is these qualities that help to ensure confidence and, in turn, lead to open, undefensive relationships where staff can enjoy the differences between people and welcome new ideas. It is in this kind of climate that residents and staff can collaborate and begin to share both responsibility and power.

BIBLIOGRAPHY

Abrams, P., Abrams, S., Humphrey, R., and Snaith, R., *Neighbourhood Care and Social Policy*, HMSO, 1989.

Allen, I., Hogg, D., and Peace, S. *Elderly People: Choice, Participation and Satisfaction* PSI 1992.

Bowlby, J., 'Self-Reliance and Some Conditions that Promote It', in Gosling, R. G. (ed), *Support, Innovation and Autonomy*, London, Tavistock Publications, 1973.

Brunel/CHI, *Value for Money*, Evaluation Working Paper 4.1, Brunel University, 1990a.

Brunel/CHI, *Ease of Implementation and Transferability*, Evaluation Working Paper 4.2, Brunel University, 1990b.

Brunel/CHI, *Consumer Satisfaction: Involving Service Users*, Evaluation Working Paper 4.3, Brunel University, 1990c.

Brunel/CHI, *Policy Statement and Guidelines on Equal Opportunities with Particular Reference to Services for Black and Minority Ethnic Groups*, Brunel University, 1990d.

Bulmer, M., *The Social Basis of Community Care*, Allen & Unwin, 1987.

Cairns, K., 'Training for Reflective Practice: Thoughts on the Education of People Who Care for Children', *The Journal of Training and Development*, Vol. 2, No. 1, 1991.

Casson, S., and George, C., *Standard Setting in Nursing Homes and Social Care Homes—The Precursor to Quality Assurance*, Social Services Department, Newcastle Upon Tyne, 1992.

CCETSW, *Setting Quality Standards for Residential Child Care: A Practical Way Forward*. A report of the Expert Group CCETSW 1992.

Centre for Environmental and Social Studies in Ageing, *Inside Quality Assurance: The IQA Action Pack*, CESSA, 1992.

Centre for Policy on Ageing, *Home Life: A Code of Practice for Residential Care*, London, CPA, 1984.

Children Act 1989

Clifford, P., Leiper, R., Lavender, T., and Pilling, S., *Assuring Quality in the Mental Health Services. The Quartz System*, RDP and Free Association Books, London, 1989.

Counsel and Care for the Elderly, *Not Such Private Places: a study of privacy and lack of privacy for residents*, Counsel and Care 1991.

Daley, T., Miller, T., and Wood, K. *Introduction to Care Planning: A Training Pack for Managers and Care Staff.* I Managers and Trainers Manual. II Workbook NISW 1992.

Davis, M., and Wallbridge, D., *Boundary and Space. An Introduction to the Work of D. W. Winnicott*, Penguin 1983.

Dawson, C., Bloch, A., and Moore, N., *Home Truths: Information About Residential Care for Elderly People*, Policy Studies Institute, 1992.

Department of Health/SSI, *Homes are For Living In*, London, HMSO, 1989a.

Department of Health and Department of Social Security, *Caring for People: Community Care in the Next Decade and Beyond*, Cm 849, London, HMSO, 1989b.

Department of Health, Social Services Inspectorate, *Caring for Quality: Guidance on Standards for Residential Homes for Elderly People*, London, HMSO, 1990a.

Department of Health, Social Services Inspectorate, *Guidance on Standards for Residential Homes for People with a Physical Disability*, London, HMSO, 1990b.

Department of Health, Social Services Inspectorate, *Guidance on Standards for the Residential Care and Needs of People with Specific Mental Health Needs*, London, HMSO, 1992a.

Department of Health, Social Services Inspectorate, *Guidance on Standards for the Residential Care Needs of People with Learning Disabilities/Mental Handicap*, London, HMSO, 1992b.

Department of Health, *The Warner Report. Choosing with Care: The Report of the Committee of Inquiry into the Selection, Development and Management of Staff in Children's Homes*, HMSO, London, 1992c.

Disabled Persons Services and Representation Act 1986

Douglas, R., and Payne, C., *Organising for Learning. Staff Development Strategies for Residential and Day Services Work. A Theoretical and Practical Guide*, National Institute for Social Work, 1988.

Dunnachie, H., 'Approaches to Quality Systems', in Kelly, D., and Warr, B., (eds), *Quality Counts: Achieving Quality in Social Care Services*, Whiting and Birch, 1992.

Elkan, R., and Kelly, D., *A Window in Homes: Links Between Residential Care Homes and the Community: A Literature Review*, Social Care Association (Education), 1990.

Faulk, L. E., 'Quality of Life Factors in Board and Care Homes for the Elderly: A Hierarchical Model', *Adult Foster Care Journal*, Vol. 2(2), Summer 1988.

Gibbs, I., and Sinclair, I. A. C., 'Checklists: Their Possible Contribution to Inspection and Quality Assurance in Old People's Homes', in Kelly, D., and Warr, B., (eds), *Quality Counts*, London, Whiting and Birch Publishers, 1992.

Goffman, E., *Stigma*, Pelican, 1968.

Guba, E. G., and Lincoln, Y., *Fourth Generation Evaluation*, Sage Publications, 1989.

Hartsock, N., 'The Feminist Standpoint', in Harding, S., and Hintikka, M. (eds), *Discovering Reality*, Reidel Pubs 1983.

Howe, E., *The Quality of Care: A Report of the Residential Staffs Inquiry*, Local Government Management Board, 1992.

Hillyard-Parker, H., Mabon, G., Payne, C., Phillipson, J., and Riley, M., *How to Manage Your Training: Developing a Training Plan*, National Institute of Social Work and the National Extension College, 1993.

Iveson, C., *Whose Life? Community Care for Old People and Their Families*, Brief Therapy Press, 1990.

Jones, S., *Police Women and Equality*, Macmillan, 1986.

Kahan, B., and Levy, A., *The Pin-Down Experience and the Protection of Children*, Report of the Staffordshire Child Care Inquiry, Staffordshire County Council, 1991.

Kelcey, C. *A Skills Self Analysis and Self Appraisal Document.* A report from the Warwickshire Independent Care Home Project. NISW 1992.

Kelly, D., 'Suspicious Minds', *Community Care*, 10 June 1993.

Kelly, D., and Warr, B., (eds), *Quality Counts*, London, Whiting and Birch Publishers, 1992.

King's Fund Centre, *An Ordinary Life*, King Edwards's Hospital Fund for London, 1980.

Lane, D. C., 'Rights, Responsibilities, Relationships and Regulations', in NISW, *Positive Answers. A Final Report of the Wagner Development Group*, London, HMSO, 1993.

Le Touze, S., and Pahl, J., *A Consumer Survey Among People with Learning Disabilities*, Centre for Health Service Studies, University of Kent, 1990.

Lewis, D., *An Information Design Audit of Information About Residential Care*, Information Design Unit, 1990.

Local Government Management Board, *Quality of Training: Guide to the Training and Development of Residential Staff*, LGMB, 1992.

Lowden, C., *How Do You Feel? An Examination of the Feelings of Elderly People Needing Care*, SCA (Education), 1992.

Mabon, G. (compiler) *An Induction Programme.* The Hampshire Independent Care Homes Project Group. NISW 1991a.

Mabon, G. (compiler) *A Policies and Procedures Handbook for Induction and Foundation Training.* NISW 1991b.

Maslow, A. H., *Motivation and Personality*, Harper Row, 1954.

McCourt-Perring, C., *The Experience of Psychiatric Hospital Closure*, Avebury, 1993.

Menzies, I., *The Functioning of Social Systems as a Defence Against Anxiety* Tavistock, London, 1970.

Miller, E. J., and Gwynne, G. V., *A Life Apart*, Tavistock Publications, 1972.

Miller, T., 'In House Training for Social Care Staff: A New Role for College Lecturers?', *Journal of Training and Development*, Vol. 2, No. 2, October 1991.

National Health Service and Community Care Act 1990.

NISW, Report of the First Eighteen Months Work of the Training for Care Staff Development Programme, NISW 1991.

NISW, *Positive Answers: Final Report of the Wagner Development Group*, London, HMSO, 1993.

Oakland, J. S., *Total Quality Management: A Practical Approach*, London DTI 1990.

Parsloe, P., and Stevenson, O., *Community Care and Empowerment*, Community Care and Joseph Rowntree Foundation, 1993.

Payne, C., and McLachlin, R., 'In Our Own Hands. The NISW/Care Weekly Guide to Self-Evaluation', *Care Weekly*, 19 May 1989.

Payne, C., 'Training for Care Staff Development Programme: Some Initial Findings' *The Journal of Training and Development* vol. 2 No. 2 1991a.

Payne, C., 'Development: The Key to Effective Training?', *The Journal of Training and Development*, Vol. 1, No. 4, 1991b.

Payne, C., 'The Evaluation Chart', *Care Weekly*, 28.2.92.

Peace, S., Kellaher, L., and Willcocks, D., *A Balanced Life? A Consumer Study of Residential Life in 100 Local Authority Old People's Homes*, Polytechnic of North London, 1982.

Peretz, E. and Payne, C. *How to Approach Staff Training in Residential Services for People with Mental Health Problems*, NISW (forthcoming).

Perring, C. A., *Residential Care and Community Care: Views of Providers, Users and Carer Organisations*, Brunel University/CHI Paper, 1991.

Phillipson, J., 'Evaluating Training Materials', *Journal of Training and Development*, Vol. 1, No. 3, 1990.

PSI, *Information for Users of Social Service Departments: Summary of Legislation and Guidance*, PSI, 1991.

PSI, *Caring in Homes Initiative: User Information Needs. A Research Proposal*, (unpublished) 1989.

Ramon, S., (ed) *Beyond Community Care: Normalisation and Integration Work.* MIND, 1991.

Roberts, S., Steele, J., and Moore, N., *Finding Out About Residential Care. Results of a Survey of Users*, PSI, 1990.

Social Care Association, *Anti-Racist Practice in Social Care: From Principles to Best Practice*, SCA, 1991.

Social Care Association (Education), *Widening Horizons: Making and Maintaining Links Between Residential Establishments and the Wider Community*, SCA, 1992a.

Social Care Association (Education), *Voluntary Links: Involving Volunteers in Developing Contacts Between Residential Establishments and the Wider Community*, SCA, 1992b.

Social Care Association (Education), *Positive Images: Developing Good Relationships Between Residential Establishments and the Wider Community*, SCA, 1992c.

Social Care Association (Education), *Giving and Taking: The Residential Home as a Community Resource*, SCA, 1992d.

Social Care Association (Education), *Communication Begins at Home: Steps Towards Developing Links Between Residential Establishments and the Wider Community*, SCA, 1992e.

Social Care Association (Education), *Blurring Boundaries: Learning from Others About Effective Links Between Residential Establishments and the Wider Community*, SCA, 1993a.

Social Care Association (Education), *Lasting Impressions: Ensuring Positive Links Between Residential Establishments and the Wider Community*, SCA, 1993b.

Standing Conference of Ethnic Minority Senior Citizens, *Ethnic Minority Senior Citizens—The Question of Policy*, SCEMSC, 1986.

Steele, J., *Information About Residential Care: The Underlying Issues*, Information Policy Working Paper 1, PSI, 1990.

Steele, J., Hinkley, R., Rowlands, I., and Moore, N., *Informing People About Social Services*, PSI, 1993.

Swarup, N., *Equal Voice: Black Communities' Views on Housing, Health and Social Services*, SSIRU, Portsmouth Polytechnic, 1992.

Utting, W., *Children in the Public Care: A Review of Residential Child Care*, HMSO, London, 1991.

Ward, L., (Ed) *Getting Better All The Time: Issues and Strategies for Ensuring Quality in Community Services for People with Mental Handicaps*. King's Fund Project paper No. 66. 1986.

Wagner, Gillian (Chairman), *Residential Care: A Positive Choice*, Report of the Independent Review of Residential Care, London, HMSO, 1988.

Weaver, T., Willcocks, D., and Kellaher, L., *The Business of Care: A Study of Private Residential Homes for Old People*, London, Polytechnic of North London, 1985.

Wenger, C., *The Supportive Network*, London, Allen & Unwin, 1984.

Willcocks, D., Peace, S., and Kellaher, L., *Private Lives in Public Places*, Tavistock Publications, 1987.

Wiseman V. Report of the Warwickshire Project (unpublished) NISW 1991.

Youll, P. J., and Aindow, S., *Black Perspectives in Service Review and Development: An Annotated Bibliography*, Brunel University, 1991.

Youll, P. J. 'The Learning Community', in Harris, et al, *Educating Social Workers*, ATSWE, 1985.

Youll, P. J., and Perring, C., *Voice and Choice: User Participation in Service Development and Evaluation*, Unpublished Paper Presented to the European Group for Public Administration, Brunel University, 1991.

APPENDICES

Appendix 1

C & E GROUP EVALUATION FIELDWORK: PROGRAMME BY PROGRAMME

1.1 Training for Care Staff Programme: NISW

1.1.a Homes Visited by Care Group

	E/EMI	MI	LD	CH	PD	DA*	Total
Total number of homes visited	12	8	3	2	2	–	27

* See key to Appendices page 231.

1.1.b Case Study Projects

	Project			
	a	b	c	Total
Sites and Agencies				
Homes visited	9	3	6	**18**
Agencies visited	–	1	7	**8**
Group Discussions and Meetings				
With staff of the care home	–	5	3	**8**
Discussions and informal meetings with residents	4	3	2	**9**
Project and Consultant Meetings				
Discussions with NISW consultant(s)	3	6	4	**13**
Observation of project meetings	10	4	3	**17**
Participation/observation in training events	3	2	1	**6**
Formal Interviews				
Managers/proprietors	4	6	6	**16**
Staff	5	10	7	**22**
Residents	–	7	6	**13**
Senior officers of the agency	–	3	6	**9**
Local SSD officers	3	3	3	**9**
Totals				
Total formal interviews	12	29	28	**69**
Total visits and meetings	29	24	26	**79**

(a) Consortium: nine private care homes + three nursing homes.
(b) Independent agency (hived off from LA) three elderly people's homes
(c) Network of nine voluntary mental health agencies

1.1.c Secondary Analysis of Projects

This involved discussions with project consultants, analysis of their records and reports together with some site visits and interviews, including follow ups. These were selected to include different care groups and sectors and to follow up particular questions or issues of interest, including links or spread to other establishments and within agencies.

	Project							
	a	b	c	d	e	f	g	Total
Site visits	2	–	2	–	2	1	1	**8**
Project meetings	–	1	2	1	2	–	–	**6**
Interviews								
Consultants	2	1	2	2	1	–	–	**8**
Managers—individual	3	–	1	–	2	2	2	**10**
Managers—group	1	–	1	1	–	–	–	**3**
Staff—individual	–	–	–	–	6	2	5	**13**
Staff-group	2	–	2	–	–	–	–	**4**
Senior officers	–	–	1	1	2	–	–	**4**
Residents	3	–	–	3	2	1	–	**9**
Total Interviews	11	1	7	7	13	5	7	**51**

(a) Two SSD run elderly peoples homes
(b) Training network for twenty-two private homes in one LA area
(c) Two SSD elderly peoples homes—extending to all homes and day centres
(d) Joint private and LA homes
(e) Sheltered housing and care establishment for Asian elders
(f) Three homes for adults with physical disability
(g) Six SSD children's homes

1.2. Inside Quality Assurance Programme: CESSA

1.2.a Homes Visited by Care Group

Care group	E/EMI	MI	LD	CH	PD	DA	Total
Total number of homes visited	8	3	2	2	2	1	18

1.2.b Case Studies of Projects

	Projects		Total
	a	b*	
Visits to the home	6	4	**10**
Group discussions/meetings			
With staff	7	2	**9**
With residents	1	–	**1**
Quality Groups	3	2	**5**
Formal interviews			
Manager	3	1	**4**
Staff	3	2	**5**
Residents	3	–	**3**
Quality Group Members (external)	4	–	**4**
SSD Officers	5	2	**7**
Total Meetings	11	5	**16**
Total Interviews	18	5	**24**

* *NB In this case no outsiders were involved in the Quality Group, feedback discussions were not held and we did not get permission to interview children, but we were able to meet the children informally with staff. In both cases there were regular discussions with consultants and full access to project records.*

(a) SSD home for elderly people
(b) SSD home for children and young people

1.2.c Secondary Analysis

This involved discussions with project consultants, analysis of their records and reports and follow-up visits and interviews after the work.

Care group	E/EMI	MI	LD	CH	PD	DA	Total
Total number of homes visited	2	3	–	2	1	–	**8**

1.2.d Homes in the Trial Round of IQA

This involved:
- site visits and interviews before, during and after the IQA pack had been tried in a sample of ten
- observation of preparatory meeting and two regional meetings during the trial
- analysis of data received in response to the CESSA's self-evaluation survey
- visits and interviews in three homes which had also been involved in another CHI project and one home which had tried BS 5750, all for elders.

	E/EMI	MI	LD	CH	PD	DA	Total
Homes selected	7	3	2	1	2	1	**16**
Home visits	6	5	3	–	4	2	**20**
Interviews*:							
Managers/senior officers	12	7	5	–	6	2	**32**
Staff/Staff Group	1 (3)	3 (1)	–	–	–	2	**6 (4)**
Residents	2	2 (1)	1 (1)	–	1	1	**9**
Quality Group Members	2	1	2	–	1	2	**8**
Total interviews	17 (3)	13 (2)	8 (1)	–	8	7	**55 (4)**

* NB Figures in brackets are group discussions with staff and residents.

1.3 Window in Homes Programme: SCA

1.3.a Homes Visited by Care Group

	E/EMI	MI	LD	CH	PD	DA	Total
Total number of homes visited	3	1	3	2	3	1	**13**

1.3.b Case Study Projects

Formal interviews with:	Numbers
Managers	1
Staff	2
Residents	4
Volunteer organisers	1
Volunteers	2
Project meetings:	
Self-advocacy group	2
Reviews	1
Meetings with consultant	2
Total Interviews	**10**
Total Meetings	**5**

1.3.c Secondary Analysis and Follow-up Visits

This involved site visits and interviews, discussions with project consultants, analysis of their records and reports.

Care Group	E/EMI	MI	LD	CH	PD	DA	Total
No. of homes	3	1	2	2	3	1	12
No. of visits	4	–	2	3	3	2	14
Interviews:*							
Consultants	3	1	2	2	3	1	12
Home managers/senior officers	3	–	2	3	2	2	12
Staff	6	–	–	(1)	3 (1)	3	12 (2)
Residents	6	–	(2)	–	4 (1)	2	12 (3)
Volunteers	–	–	–	–	1	–	1
Externals	–	–	1	–	–	–	1
Total interviews	18	1	5 (2)	5 (1)	13 (2)	8	50 (5)

* Interviews and discussions with staff teams and groups of residents marked in brackets.

1.4 Information for Users of Social Services Programme: PSI

1.4.a Fieldwork undertaken
- case studies of two pilot projects
- outline study of four pilot projects
- observation of Consultative Group meetings (four + two day workshop)
- observation of Programme meetings/seminars
- analysis of project records and materials
- discussions with consultants

1.4.b Case Studies and Visits to Pilot SSDS

	Case Study Pilots			Other Pilot SSDS
	a	b	c	
Visits and observation of project meetings	3	2	$1\frac{1}{2}$ days	3
Interviews:				
Senior SSD Personnel	4	3	2	
Information and research officers	2	–	1	
Project workers	5	–	2	
Discussions with PSI Consultant	4	–	2	2

Analysis of Local Authority policy documents, information materials

Additional Interviews:
SSD information officers (3)
Physical disability information project (1)
Commercial information systems specialist (1)

(a) Shire authority: urban population
(b) Metropolitan authority
(c) Shire authority NW: dispersed and rural population

1.5 'Home Truths': Information about Residential Care for Elderly People'

1.5.a Work undertaken

- Questionnaire survey of sample of people who attended the CHI conferences

Sample	206
Responses from purchasers	15
Responses from non-purchasers	45
Total	60
(Response Rate	29%)

- Questionnaire survey of sample of direct purchasers selected to include senior officers, inspectors and all establishments

Sample	49
Responses	16
(Response rate	32%)

- Interviews with and commentaries from

Managers, staff, residents, carers in six homes	17
Individual purchasers	5
Representatives: organisations for elderly people and their carers	11

Total no. of interviews	**33**

Appendix 2

AGENCIES AND ORGANISATIONS INTERVIEWED OR CONSULTED BY THE C & E GROUP

Care and Interest Groups	Organisations
Elders	Age Concern *Standing Conference of Ethnic Minority Senior Citizens Centre for Policy on Ageing *Pensioners' Link Help the Aged Alzheimer's Disease Society Methodist Homes for the Aged Asian Sheltered Residential Association
Mental Health	National Schizophrenia Fellowship—NSF Association of Therapeutic Communities MENCAP *MINDLINK Afro-Caribbean Mental Health Association—ACMHA Richmond Fellowship Mental Aftercare Association—MACA
Learning Disabilities	*People First Values Into Action Mencap Association for Residential Care—ARC
Physical Disability/ Sensory Impairment	Royal National Institute for the Deaf—RNID Royal National Institute for the Blind—RNIB Spastics Society Multiple Sclerosis Society *Disability Alliance *Royal Association for Disability and Rehabilitation Oxford Disability Information Project *CHOICE, London Borough of Barnet
Drug/Alcohol	Standing Conference on Drug Abuse—SCODA Alcohol Concern

Children and Young People	London Boroughs Regional Children's Planning Committee National Council of Voluntary Child Care Organisations Voice of the Child in Care *National Association of Young People in Care—NAYPIC National Children's Bureau
Care Home Associations	Dorset Care Homes Association Hampshire Residential Care Homes Association
Housing Associations	National Federation of Housing Associations
Carers/Relatives	Carers National Association—CNA Relatives Association
Unions	National and Local Government Officers Association—NALGO
Black and Ethnic Minority Interests	Race Equality Unit (NISW)
HIV/AIDS	Waverley Trust, Edinburgh

* User/user-run organisations

Appendix 3

ANALYSIS OF EVALUATION DATA

The Different Levels and Types of Evaluation

Case Studies

These were treated as studies in their own right. Interviews, records of visits, meetings and so on were analysed to produce a detailed feedback report including an analytical description of the work and a critical commentary. These were discussed first with Programme consultants and participants and then with Programme Managers. These were used to inform our overall analysis. Data from interviews (but not informal observations and discussions) were also analysed as part of the overall interview set for the relevant Programme.

Interviews

All the interviews, including those with managers and senior officers where we used a semi-structured schedule, allowed for open ended responses. A key problem in analysing qualitative information is to cover the range and check impressions for accuracy and weight, while doing justice to the depth and detail of what people had to say. Traditional statistical techniques would have been quite inappropriate, and unhelpful, in analysing the experiences and perspectives of the range of people involved or affected by the work.

We used a text analysis programme—Textbase Alpha (by Sommerland and Kristensen, University of Aarhus, Denmark)—which has recently been developed for computer-assisted analysis of qualitative data. This allows narrative texts, such as interviews and other records, to be post-coded by the researcher and sorted to produce files on particular questions, themes and relationships between different areas of interest. We found this method to be feasible and valuable for research of this type, attemping, as it did, to combine qualitative and detailed data with a wide scope of coverage. Where numbers of interviews were smaller, as in the PSI Programme, it was not used.

Data base

The initial aim was to collect information about establishments involved in projects in order to provide a general profile and indicators of service quality and change. Questionnaires were to be completed by consultants for each home in which they were doing detailed work, including information gathering for Programme purposes. This needed to be done at an early stage, before development work, if it was to provide indicators or evidence of change linked to the work.

In the event, fifty-three questionnaires were returned out of a total of ninety homes involved in project work of this type (i.e. excluding homes involved in early pilots, the IQA independent trial sites, networks or where no active project plans were developed). Most were not completed at an early stage due to uncertainties and delays in securing access and agreement in projects by Programmes. The database could not be used to assess change but it did provide reliable background information about the range of homes, their relative stability, staffing profiles, ethnicity, quality indicators. The information was loaded into a computer programme Statistical Package for the Social Sciences, for analysis (SPSS.PC).

The more statistical data was pre-coded—for example, numbers of residents and staff—and more qualitative data was post-coded, as far as possible, according to relevant categories, so that it could be analysed using SPSS.PC. This package is able to handle a limited amount of qualitative data and was useful for checking our overall impressions of context and practice in the homes involved.

Analysis of Programme and Project Records

Since we could not visit all projects and interview all the people involved, secondary analysis was important to give a greater scope and coverage to the evaluation. Consultants from selected projects shared their detailed records with us and these were read and compared to highlight recurring issues of interest in the Programme. In particular, the records were analysed for information about the processes involved, the timing and sequence of activities, who carried out the work and the nature of the relationship between participants. The outcomes of the projects were considered in relation to the original objectives of the work and whether these had been fulfilled.

Analysis of IQA Questionnaires

In the trial of the prototype IQA pack, the Programme researchers sent out short questionnaires to the 107 homes and agencies participating. These asked eight questions about reasons for involvement, the experience and the impact of the review. The CESSA team kindly allowed us to use the responses to re-analyse and this proved useful for comparison and giving a broader base to our interviews in sample sites.

Forty-seven questionnaires were returned. We categorised and sorted the main types of responses and these were used to formulate our commentary in Chapter 3.

Questionnaire Survey of PSI Work

The booklet *Home Truths* was evaluated by a short postal questionnaire survey of purchasers and by interviews with personnel in selected homes. The survey returns were numerically small and could be analysed question by question.

Confidentiality

Interview notes or tapes and questionnaires were entered onto the computer anonymously but were coded so that we could identify patterns across projects, care groups, local authorities and so on.

Appendix 4

PROGRAMME COVERAGE OF AGENCIES AND RESIDENTIAL ESTABLISHMENTS

Programmes ran a series of projects, each of which involved one or more care establishments. Several projects involved more than one agency.

4.1 Total CHI Coverage

4.1.a Total Number of Homes Participating in Programmes

		Sector			Care Group*						
Projects	Total	P	V	St	E	EMI	MI	LD	PD	DA	CH
SCA	47	2	25	20	12	1	6	15	3	1	7
NISW	104	54	17	33	71	1	13	8	3	–	11
CESSA	109	23	21	60	61	10	12	6	9	3	3
Totals	260	79	63	113	144	12	31	29	15	4	21

* See key to Appendices page 231.

4.1.b Agencies Involved by Programme

Programme	LA areas included	Care Assns	Vol Orgs	Other Orgs	Network projects	Non-home based projects eg evaluation	Total No of projects*
NISW	18	1	12	1	4	4	23
CESSA	54	1	13	–	1	–	109
SCA	22	–	18	–	–	–	29
PSI—Info Guidelines	12	–	–	1	–	6	6

* Projects varied in the number of homes or agencies involved.

4.2 Summary of Data on CESSA Projects

4.2.a Total Number of Homes Involved

Total	Sector				Care Group							
	P	V	St	NK	E	EMI	MI	LD	C/YP	PD	DA	NK
109	23	21	60	5	61	10	12	6	3	9	3	5

4.2.b Agencies Involved

	Total LAs	Total Agencies	Care Assns	Vol Agencies	Other (Housing Assns)
Total*	54	14	1	9	4

Some homes were involved in more than one round and different homes from the same agency/local authority were involved in development and trial rounds.

4.2.c Homes in Trial of IQA Pack by Size

No. of beds	0-9	10-19	20-29	30-39	40+	NK
No. of homes	5	12	20	21	32	7

4.3 Summary Data on SCA Projects

4.3.a Total Number of Homes Involved by Sector and Care Group

	Total No of homes	Sector			Care Group						
		P	V	St	E	EMI	MI	LD	C/YP	PD	DA
Pilot	10	1	2	7	2	–	2	2	3	1	–
Main projects	37	1	23	13	10	1	4	15*	4	2	1
	47	2	25	20	12	1	6	17	7	3	1

* This total includes two homes for people with learning disabilities and sensory impairment.

4.3.b Homes in Main Projects by Size

No. of beds	0-9	10-19	20-29	30-39	40+	NK	TOT
No. of homes	13	7	4	6	4	3	37

4.4 Summary Data on NISW Projects

4.4.a Total Number of Homes Involved

		Sector			Care Group					
	T	P	V	S	E	EMI	MI	LD	CH	PD
Total	104	54	17	33	68	1	13	8	11	3

4.4.b Training Project Types

Type of Project	No. of:—			No. of Homes/Care Group						
	Project Nos	Agencies	LAs	E/EMI	MI	LD	CH	PD	DA
Home based	14	8	12	28	2	8	11	3	–
Network/ Consortia	4	8	3	41	11	–	–	–	–
Evaluation:									
Training Materials	1	–	–			N/A			
Local Authority Training Strategy/Course	2*	–	2			N/A			
Role of Training Resource Centres	2	–	2			N/A			
NVQ Developments	2*	–	2			N/A			

* Overlap with home-based projects

KEY TO APPENDICES

CH	Children and Young People
DA	Drug or Alcohol Problems
E	Elders
EMI	Elders with Dementia
LD	Learning Disability
MI	Mental Illness
NK	Not Known
P	Private Homes
PD	Physical Disability
S	Statutory Agencies
V	Voluntary Agencies

GLOSSARY

CCETSW	Central Council for Education and Training in Social Work
C & E Group	The Coordination and Evaluation Group of the Caring in Homes Initiative
CEPPP	Centre for the Evaluation of Public Policy and Practice, Brunel University
CESSA	Centre for the Environmental and Social Studies of Ageing, University of North London
CHI	Caring in Homes Initiative
CHOICE	Case Management Service, Barnet for people with disabilities
DOH	Department of Health
IQA	Inside Quality Assurance
LA	Local Authority
NAYPIC	National Association of Young People in Care
NCVCCO	National Council for Voluntary Child Care Organisations
NDIP	National Disability Information Project
NHS	National Health Service
NISW	National Institute for Social Work
NVQ	National Vocational Qualification
PNL	Polytechnic of North London (now University of North London)
Programme	The research Programmes run by the Caring in Homes agencies
PSI	Policy Studies Institute
REU	Race Equality Unit
SCA	Social Care Association
SCA (Education)	Social Care Assocation (Education)
SCEMSC	Standing Conference on Ethnic Minority Senior Citizens
SCODA	Standing Conference on Drug Abuse
SSI	Social Services Inspectorate
WDG	Post Wagner Development Group
VOCC	Voice for the Child in Care

Printed in the United Kingdom for HMSO
Dd296416 11/93 C20 G531 10170